WINGS OF POWER

WINGS OF POWER

Progressive Yoga Relaxation

Margrit Segesman

Thorough absorption of all problems
by the subconscious leaves the mind
free to attend fully to the art of
dynamic creative living.

Harper & Row, Publishers
New York, Evanston, San Francisco, London

First published in Australia by Hill of Content Publishing Company Pty. Ltd.

FIRST U.S. EDITION

Library of Congress Cataloging in Publication Data
Segesman, Margrit.
  Wings of power; progressive yoga relaxation.
  1. Yoga, Hatha.   2. Relaxation.   I. Title.
RA781.7.S433 1974   613.7   74-1855
ISBN 0-06-013833-5

Foreword

A Student Writes

The taxi stopped. It rushed me during a lunch hour to an old fashioned villa in Melbourne's Queens Road and one of my first yoga lessons. Sitting on the steps in the bright sunshine Margrit Segesman welcomed me, a bowl of fruit salad in one hand, and invited me to sit with her while she finished eating. This ordinary scene has stayed with me in clarity and detail down the years. No doubt it was a moment consciously lived; the warm sunshine, peaceful road, luxury of escape from weekday business and the friendly, easy circumstance of my encounter with this remarkable personality who was to have such a profound effect upon my life.

Margrit Segesman was then, and still is, a powerful combination of highly intellectual and cultured mind, cosmopolitan sophistication and the mystique of one who studied for many years with a Guru in the seclusion of the Himalayas. Her mission in life is to teach.

She believes that there exists within man a power which he can use as wings to explore new dimensions of freedom and self development. She believes also that there is a way by which people can free themselves from anxieties, fears, tensions and 'hang-ups', compulsions and addictions and achieve fulfilment of themselves by using all the potentialities of their unlimited minds.

Since those early days in Queens Road in 1955, Margrit Segesman has built up the finest school of yoga in Australia where thousands of students have now studied with her the esoteric teachings and methods of Progressive Yoga Relaxation.

At the request of many of her former and present students and in answer to an inner bidding, Margrit Segesman has now summed up her wide experience, particularly in yoga relaxation which she regards as a pre-requisite to successful progress in the science of yoga and all its implications and applicability to our everyday lives.

To ensure the anonymity of people
concerned in the case histories
names and identities of most have
been altered.

Contents

Acknowledgement

I would like to acknowledge with deep gratitude the help and contributions of my staff, especially June Bingham, Eve Degen, Susan Gabor and Bianca McCullough who made it possible for me to draw on their individual talents in compiling and clarifying such a large volume of teaching material.

I would also like to thank Ginia Roesler and Gina Paxton who, as students over many years, have given me their views and experiences regarding certain techniques.

And I am grateful to the large body of students of the Gita School of Yoga with whom I have worked and grown in knowledge.

Margrit Segesman.

Preface

I believe in Evolution; in the eventual spiritualisation of man and the whole Universe; that there is a divine plan and that the Universe is not just an incidental concurrence of atoms, but is planned to minute detail.

There exists within man the power to contact the universal forces by which he is capable of doing anything that he may aspire to do or be. This book sets out to explain the tuning in to the descending forces, giving man wings to ascend to unimaginable heights there to explore the fullness of his liberation.

I also believe in prevention rather than healing. The idea of the ancient Chinese of paying the doctor when healthy and fit and making him pay in the case of sickness, always seems so much more reasonable than our way.

Progressive Yoga Relaxation is one of the best methods of keeping fit by clearing out of the subconsciousness what could cause hypertension now and sickness in the future.

With a positive attitude, life is limitless in its magnitude. Life is exciting; it should be a continuous adventure. Hidden deep in every human being are millions of wonderful new ideas waiting impatiently to be discovered. It does not matter whether it is a world shaking idea or the arranging of a miniature garden in a one room apartment.

A day without improvement is a day lost. From the moment of opening one's eyes in the morning until closing them in sleep at night, there should be a great love for life, willingness to meet new people, make new friends, consider new ideas and invite the expansion of universal awareness. To be in love with life is to enjoy all the heart warming, insignificant happenings of every ordinary day.

If you are discontented with your life — change it! Do not plod on letting the unhappiness seep deeper and deeper into your soul. Man is the architect of his own life. Every single human being has the free will to do what he wants with himself; this is his glorious birthright, regardless of whether he was born in the slums or with a silver spoon in his mouth. Even those born crippled or handicapped can still shape their lives. There are few without the necessary intellectual faculties to learn something new or go to school or attend an institution for educating and training physically or mentally handicapped people. What you need is the determination to use every little bit of what you have.

Get to know more about yourself; alter the blue-print of your self image. Go ahead! And do not stop until the goal — the understanding of yourself — is reached. This will make you more perceptive of others and, in turn, increase your personal dynamism and creative living.

M.S.

Stanza

Listen, O worker in the furthest world,
   to the rhythm of the times,
Note the pulsation in the heart,
   of that which is Divine,
Retire into the silence,
   and attune yourself unto the Whole.
Then venture forth,
Establish the right rhythm;
Bring order to the forms of life,
Which must express the Plan of Deity.

For the Blessed One, release is found in work,
He must display his knowledge
   of the Plan by the sounding of those words,
Which will evoke the Builders of the forms,
   and thus create the new.

                              from the Book of Dzyan.*

*The age of the Book of Dzyan is unknown. It is said to
contain the secret wisdom of the past, present and future of
mankind, and is written in Senzar, a language of crypts and
symbols. In the second half of last century H. P. Blavatsky
was fortunate to come across it in Tibet and was given per-
mission to translate part of it into English. The Stanzas have
a haunting beauty of their own and a sacred quality which
makes them strangely uplifting.

Introduction

In my late teens, after the death of my fiance, and childhood sweetheart, I contracted a virulent form of tuberculosis. The doctors gave me very small chance of survival. I wanted to stay in the hospital of my small home town in Switzerland, to be near my family, but being contagious, I was sent to a special sanatorium in the Alps. For many years I left the place only when I had to undergo one of several operations in Berne. Drugs to cure T.B. had not yet been discovered and the treatment consisted mostly of surgery; the rest depended on fresh air and one's own resistance.

Life in the sanatorium was extremely unreal. For many it became idle and boring. There was, of course, the daily routine and the treatment; but for the remainder of the day we were supposed to rest. A kind of social life prevailed. Most of the patients lapsed into a trivial pattern of visiting each other, playing chess, bridge, poker, or other games; and then there were the endless discussions about all and everything.

In such a small and restricted community people fell in and out of love, or stayed together; this was accepted, but there was an unwritten law that parting had to be undramatic for the public. Past lovers had to be socially friendly, if they wanted to stay in the group.

The first few weeks I was not allowed visitors, as the doctors were establishing my left side pneumothorax (a surgical treatment to reduce the breathing activity of one side of the lungs to a bare minimum, thereby giving the lesions a chance to close and heal). This suited me very well as I did not feel like communicating. I was numb with despair about my loss and the illness, but even more hurt by the strange attitude of my father. He had always been a health fanatic and he hated sickness like a personal enemy. When he heard the news about me he refused to believe it, but I knew it was only a sort of escape from reality, as I had seen the fear and repulsion in his eyes and the vision haunted me.

As long as I can remember I had admired and worshipped my father and now, when I needed him most, he did not even write to me.

I managed to accept my condition and bring some order in my life. Whenever I was well enough I would study persevering with a curriculum in philosophy. It was in the first half year of my stay at the sanatorium that they started experimenting with double pneumothoraxes. I had made no progress so far, so I was one of the first on the list. Before the second pneumothorax could begin, some adherences of the lungs to the pleura had to be cauterised.

At last it was all over and I had a double pneumothorax. For weeks I could only breathe sitting up in bed and, as I was too breathless to study, the days dragged; but the nights were worse. In spite of the heavy sedation, after only a few hours I would wake up gasping for air, soaked in cold sweat and a feeling that a relentless force was squeezing my lungs until, half demented with terror, I could stand it no longer and would ring for the night nurse.

She treated me like a naughty child and she would address me as 'we', saying: 'Are we breathless again? Can we not manage to be alone?' and so on. I resented this kind of talk bitterly, but anything was better than being alone with that dreadful fear of suffocation. The only subject of interest for the nurse was her fiance, whom I did not know, but I stalled her departure with questions about him, having a deep down sense of degradation about my insincerity.

Then, at last, dawn would come; every dawn being a gift of another day. Oh, those thousands of dawns — incredibly beautiful, each different; in winter so gentle and translucent that you never quite knew when they had started; in summer explosions of light, pregnant with the promise of long, sunny days, changing into symphonies of colour in spring and autumn.

In these times of isolation I learned a lot about human relationships and especially about fear and tension. I started to analyse fear, to observe it in myself and in others and slowly I could see the same pattern emerge in everyone; physical contraction of the diaphragm, butterflies, squaring of the shoulders, stiffening of the neck and back of the head, biting the teeth together and tensing of the whole body. Mentally, there was the narrowing of the mind to one point, focusing on one subject only — the particular fear.

When I was sure of my observations, I wrote them all down. I started to undo the tension backwards, first to make the whole body easy and then one part after the other. It took me a long time because I was much too anxious to succeed, but it was very good for me as it captured my mind. No book on relaxation had been written, because relaxation, as a technique, was unknown at that time.

Firstly, I used this technique of relaxation only in the night, when I woke up stiff with fear. It worked, and soon I did not need the night nurse any more. Then I relaxed before injections and all the other painful treatments. With time I even used relaxation during the refilling of the pneumothorax, and instead of soporifics at night. The other patients noticed the change in my behaviour because I seemed more at ease, so I told some of them about the technique and several were soon able to do it. To the very sick ones I gave soft spoken suggestions and that technique was also effective.

But all the time I had an uneasy feeling at the back of my mind. I knew there was more to it — this whole experiment was only fragmentary. I went over and over my experiences, I looked at it from every angle and at last I realised —

There are two kinds of tension:
1 Tension through will to create.
2 Tension through fear.

The first kind of tension is brought on voluntarily through the will to create and uses universal force positively. The freer of 'hangups' a person is, the stronger the creative tension becomes. The second kind of tension is compulsory and is triggered off by fear and it uses universal force negatively. The more complexes, traumas, and anxiety a person has, the stronger becomes the negative power of tension through fear.

It was like magic. The understanding of the two different tensions helped me to get rid of fear of tuberculosis and my health improved extraordinarily. Until now I had responded very little to all the treatments, surgery included, but from that moment, I just went ahead.

I wanted to discuss my experience with fear and positive thinking with doctors, but they worked too hard to have time to listen long enough. Each thought I was too much alone and they unanimously recommended more social activity.

Whenever I started talking about it with the other patients, it developed into one of those unending discussions. So I kept it all to myself and it was the great adventure of my life, using it daily, realising I was the architect of my life, be it success or failure.

It was during this time that I had my first spiritual experience and practically overnight I changed from an agnostic to a believer.

By now I was allowed to be up for dinner and the evening entertainment; films, lectures, discussions and an occasional dance. I enjoyed these evenings tremendously, especially the experience of being with larger groups of people, as I did not at all care for visiting and playing cards.

The rest of the day I kept to a schedule; studying philosophy in the morning, reading modern literature during the siesta and doing things with my hands before dinner. I had made some animals out of cloth for my small cousins. It was, at that time, a completely new idea. One of the patients was a publisher of German magazines and he ordered the models and instructions for a whole magazine of rag animals. The next thing he wanted was a magazine of standard doll's clothing, knitted and sewn. That led to knitted models for people. I sent photographs and descriptions of my models to firms all over Europe and soon I had more orders than I could deliver. When I got bored, I started designing curtain and furniture material with Armand, a French art student, who had only a slight infection. We were an ideal team; he designed my ideas much better than I could. We earned good money, gained the approval and respect of the doctors and the patients; most important for me was the proof of my theory on success and failure.

After Armand left I continued designing for a while, but it was not the same without him and I missed him terribly.

A school friend asked me to do research work for his thesis on primitive North Italian painters and I was very glad for the change. Then another friend needed some help for his thesis on the old laws of Burgundy. I then wrote a few articles which were printed, but I somehow felt not enough in contact with the world and put writing aside for the time being.

And so the years went by and at last I was declared cured; but I was left with only one fourth of normal breathing capacity. I was a stranger to my family and the change from the high altitude to the low land gave me a very noticeable wheezing-breath, which seemed to irritate my parents, and disturbed most people. I missed the steady routine of the sanatorium. I felt a freak; a twenty-five year old with the experiences and dreams of a teenager. The world, also, had changed drastically, prosperity had given way to depression, and everyone seemed afraid and tense.

When my favourite aunt and uncle invited me on a world tour I accepted with pleasure, especially as it entailed a job. I had to keep Aunt Rolande company during my Uncle Henry's explorations. He was interested in just about everything and no temple was too far off the beaten track and no ruin too insignificant; he had to see it all.

They were very happily married, but my aunt could not share his enthusiasm as her fastidiousness prevented her from enjoying the rougher parts of the trip. She preferred reading travelogues in the comfort of her room and she was so well versed that she was a match in knowledge for my uncle. I typed uncle's travel notes and when my aunt saw my eagerness she let me go with him and we had a marvellous time together. They were lovely; they never seemed to notice my shortness of breath and they never thought things could be too much for me. My uncle taught me some breathing exercises, which were a great help, and I showed them relaxation. We had a fascinating time; I lost the feeling of having been cheated out of the best years of my life.

After our return I had a letter from Armand in Paris. By now he was married, and he and his wife invited me to visit them. I went, and made up my mind to stay and look for work. A fashion house for knitted models, with whom I already had a connection, gave me a position in its salon. In my spare time I worked freelance with Armand and Janine.

We had interesting weekends together in the country around Paris.

Armand and Janine became the parents of twins, a girl and a boy; they would have liked to see me married and settled, but I was happy as I was. I became more and more involved with the fast living crowd of the haute couture and I fell passionately in love with a Polish diplomat. I had a wonderful, if hectic life; the only flaw was his jealousy. He was jealous of everyone and everything. At first I was quite flattered, but that soon wore off and it became the cause of constant quarrels. He wanted me to give up my job, my friends, and my pets; I had to tell him where I would be at any given time of the day. He decided what I should wear, in fact he would have liked to control my whole life. At last I could stand it no longer; I was becoming a nervous wreck, and, like a coward, I sneaked away without an explanation.

I had always wanted to invite my Aunt Rolande and Uncle Henry for another world tour. I think they guessed my problem, but they never said a word and we had an even better time than before because I had played with the idea of this trip for many months and the travel agency did their very best.

I wrote my fiance and explained to him that I could not go on as I could not enter a marriage without mutual trust.

On my return to Paris he was gone; he had been transferred to another country and everything was as before, but I could not settle. I was bored, I missed him and was looking for a more meaningful life.

It was on a long weekend in Switzerland that I happened to mention my experiences about relaxation and expansion of consciousness to Professor C. G. Jung. He suggested I take up the study of Yoga.

Following his advice I went to the national library and was astonished at how many different Yogas existed. First, I studied *The Science of Breath* by Yogi Ramacharaka [Fowler (L.N.) and Company Limited]. It was a revelation. I practised the new knowledge avidly and, after a few months, my breathing technique had improved so much that my affliction was not noticeable anymore.

I gave up all extra work and devoted my free time to the study of Yoga. Because I found it so absorbing, I stayed at home more and more in the evenings and on the weekends. It was all very fascinating; there were so many different Yogas, so much contradiction, that I became quite confused. As I continued it began to make sense. After a time my interest focused on Raja Yoga, also called the Yoga of the Kings, and Hatha Yoga.

Raja Yoga is a man's union with the highest plane. It is a discipline of the mind; a system of mental and ethical training to develop will power and concentration through the understanding that the innermost soul is the ruler. From this, therefore, proceeds the fact that every human being is his own master — the ruler of his own destiny. This demands detachment from the egocentric personality; discrimination between truth and fantasy. Once illusion has been overcome, the individual is in control of forces whose existence are unknown to the average man.

Hatha Yoga consists of physical exercises and breathing techniques. It works on the metabolism and on the nervous system; it is very invigorating. Hatha Yoga uses physical means for spiritual self-development. It is a helpful prelude and assistant to Raja Yoga.

Then the war broke out and I returned to my family. We all thought the war would end in no time, but it dragged on. I took a flat and joined a welfare organisation to help the families of soldiers who were in the border guard. Switzerland was neutral, but was surrounded by countries at war with each other.

We had bicycles as there was petrol only for industry. I caught a bad infection of the throat, but as we were understaffed I continued working till I was hospitalized with a crippling attack of arthritis. As soon as I could walk on sticks I resumed work, but slowly I became worse in spite of all the treatment.

Relaxation helped me to cope with the excruciating pain, but it came as a great shock when I was told that it was only a matter of one or two years and I would not be able to walk any more. As soon as the war was over, I started my pilgrimage in search of a cure. Wherever I went the diagnosis was the same; incurable, getting progressively worse.

I was frantic and tried everything I read or heard of; among other things I fasted for thirty-seven days. It helped a bit, but I lost so much weight I had to stop before my intentional fifty days. After having put on some weight I began a real 'horse-cure' — sauna. I would have a bath as hot as I could possibly stand and then I would go and roll in the snow. This procedure I repeated three times at about four in the morning as I did not want to be seen. Perhaps it could have cured me, but I got pneumonia and I had to battle hard to survive.

Chastened and very weak, I decided to give up forceful things and try psychoanalysis as I had read about psychosomatic diseases. By now I had reached a sort of grim humour. I went to one psychoanalyst after the other, but they all said the same thing, that I was sane and did not need to be analysed; I just had to accept my illness. As I was not ready to do this, I had to find something else; and so, at last, I started to work on myself. When I tried to analyse myself I became very tense and frustrated and had to do relaxation for longer and longer periods to get rid of the strain, until, at last, I did only relaxation.

I continued for a few weeks and had what I then thought were queer experiences, my legs and arms jerked as sometimes happens before going to sleep, then my whole body would tremble, or a deep sadness would come over me and I would cry helplessly without knowing why. This was rather surprising as I had been brought up not to cry. I also relived several very early childhood happenings and experienced almost unbearable strain. Another time I had a feeling of floating weightlessly in the sky. As different as these experiences were, they had one thing in common — I always felt physically and mentally better afterwards.

One day during relaxation, in a state of timelessness, I experienced love of God which ended all my searchings for an aim in life. Floating on a sea of light I felt the vibration of love, the highest vibration existing.

Here I will try to do the impossible — to explain spiritual experiences through intellectual language.

Love is the foundation of all things, it is the soul of all forms, it is the quintessence of the universal mind — the *anima-mundi*.

Love is the magnetic force which holds the world together.

Love is responsible for Creation and is the reason for its maintenance.

Love is the greatest existing force, which not only creates, but also binds and sustains.

Love is our will to be; without it the world would disintegrate into the void, into nothingness.

Love is a call and it evokes an answer.

Love is attraction and responsible for all relationships.

Love overcomes all differences: It can bind opposites and act as a mediator.

Love gives understanding, it is the bridging force between the kingdoms of nature.

Without love we would not be able to stand this life and continue living.

Love is the greatest, the most wonderful, the most splendid, the most magnificent thing.

I was so elated that it took me by surprise when I realised I was moving about without my sticks.

I had known for a few years that my life was too superficial, that I had to do more with it; that one's life is only as good as the good it brings to other people. I had been very reluctant to leave the world of fashion where I was accepted and at home. Now, with deliberate use of all the transcendental effect of Yoga Relaxation, I shed my last deep hidden fears and gained the courage to do what I felt in my conscience was the only right thing. I had to break away from the conventional way of life and venture out into the unknown. I had to give up this self-centredness, expand, and live more altruistically. Once I had thought this through I went ahead and made contact with a few Yoga centres (ashrams) in India; three of them invited me to join them.

My family opposed my going to India and my father expressed their opinion when he said: 'One goes to India to bring them Christianity, not to learn their heathen ways'. I did not mention my project any more; I just did all the preparation, and one day I left; the people assuming I was on a long holiday. My friends had told me I was much too sophisticated to be able to live in a primitive way. To get used to hardship I decided to hitch-hike leisurely to India. Here, I must admit, if I had known the hardship and the various disappointments ahead, I doubt if I would have gone.

It was difficult as very few people had done this trip up to that time; but in a funny sort of way it was the easiest time of my life. I am glad I did it, the experience makes me understand the wandering young people of today. There is a strange timelessness in wandering, living for the present only, without responsibility, no past, no future. It is easy to talk and communicate with everyone, to say things you would normally not mention, as you reveal too much of yourself; but what does it matter, you will never come across that person again; tomorrow you will be far away in a new place meeting other strangers but for a short time you feel loved and at ease. You have practically no possessions, only the few things you are ready to carry.

Once in India I visited several ashrams and stayed in one in northern India. This ashram was really a complete town and the only law was the guru, but he was rarely there as he was very old and frail and one received few instructions. I decided to look for a guru with only a few students and, with the help of a wandering yogi, my search ended. I found my guru living in a cave, and for years I knew nothing else but meditation, Raja Yoga, Hatha Yoga, the intense practices of Kriya and Tantra, study of cosmology and evolution. The first few months were the hardest. I nearly lost my mind and I still do not know which was more difficult to bear — the utter loneliness or the crushing grandeur of the Himalayan Ranges. Slowly I settled in deep contentment.

I lost count of the years as my meditation became deeper and I had only one desire — to stay with my guru. He was the personification of love for me, but deep down I knew that some day I would have to leave and teach. One day, out of the blue, my guru told me he would go further from civilisation, higher up the mountains, and I had to go back to the western world.

All the years with my guru I had a clean shaven head and I wore the habit of a swami. I looked like a man as I weighed only six stone. Before leaving India and returning to the western civilisation I had to fill out a bit and let my hair grow.

In due time I lost my ascetic look and as soon as my straight, short hair could take a perm I sailed for Melbourne as I felt attracted to Australia.

It took a few weeks to polish up my rusty school English. As I intended to teach free of charge, I needed a source of income and I found work as a sales-manageress. The people I met knew very little about Relaxation, Yoga and Positive Thinking and most considered me a sort of crackpot.

I had only a few, irregular students till John joined up. He was a very popular, dynamic radio-announcer; hard working, hard playing. He immediately understood the power of the mind and a long cherished innovation was at last introduced in his main program. His long standing old dermatitis disappeared practically overnight.

His enthusiasm brought me a lot of his friends, and one of them, a psychoanalyst, suggested full-time teaching and charging a minimal fee. I took his advice after my first radio interview.

There was such a response that I had to give up my job and devote myself entirely to the teaching of healthy, positive living with only the sky as a limit.

Till I had well trained teachers I taught alone. The school has grown steadily and up to the time of writing over thirty thousand students have attended. There are now fourteen teachers at the Gita School and hundreds, all over the world, teaching the unlimited power of the human mind.

Man's Place in Evolution

There is a great deal of controversy in regard to the doctrine of spiritual evolution, reincarnation and karma; yet the same people who doubt spiritual evolution accept without query the fact of physical evolution — the development of the body from previous forms, participation in a slow, perpetual transformation of all living things. These people consider the story of evolution as part of history, following it from primeval humanity to modern civilization.

So it is unimportant whether evolution is observed through the laws of inheritance, considering every child as slightly more evolved than its parents and holding ancestors responsible for all distinguishing features in character, physiognomy and habits, or from the view point of those who favour the theory of karma and reincarnation with each soul progressing through every new life and taking full responsibility for its own character traits. The difference is only a matter of degree.

There are those who vaguely think of reincarnation as having something to do with trans-migration, that is, a soul's descent at the time of death into the body of an animal. Others are petrified by the mistaken idea that reincarnation means the eternal wheel of human rebirth *ad infinitum,* without let-up — a hopeless concept. Then there are those extreme opposites who, having grasped the principle of spiritual emancipation, imagine that through some *tour-de-force* they can magically twist the arm of karma and thereby overcome the necessity to reincarnate after their present existence. Only deep, all embracing love brings earthly karma to an end.

Karma is the law of cause and effect, of action and reaction, its working cannot be evaded, no prayer can change its course.

Karma is action both in the religious and worldly sense; it is the law of attraction and repulsion. Like attracts like — the law is as simple as that. Whatever we desire most strongly we will get. If we desire and concentrate on becoming loving in temperament, love will come from everywhere to meet us. If, on the other hand, we give out rejection and hatred we will suffer rejection and hatred in return.

Life and karma can be compared to a large river. Everyone has to travel along it, but each is free to choose his own tempo and mode of locomotion. We may travel in the middle of the river on a luxury boat, absorbed in daily pleasures; we may ride in a speedboat, interested only in the tempo and the desire to go ahead faster than anyone else; or we may prefer a canoe, pausing wherever the shore looks inviting, or sailing along using the winds of chance to progress. We may swim, depending on our own strength or again ride with friends in a houseboat. The choice is unlimited from birth until death, but travel we must down the river.

The Creator's gift to his children is free will and karma is the direct descendant of free will. It is our decision, how we wish to apply this free will — by following the voice of the soul, or the voice of the personality; by striving for spiritual progress, or the satisfaction of our personal desires. Often we will find it very difficult to discriminate between the two. There is a simple test we should ask ourselves, 'Will it hurt anyone?' — remembering that sometimes we have to hurt, as when saying 'No' to a child. Then the test is: 'Do I personally benefit by it?' If you are still in doubt, follow your instinct and remember, if you were infallible, you could not learn anything more on earth and you would not be here! We only learn through repeatedly making the same mistakes. It is helpful to cultivate a positive attitude. Rather than smother ourselves in useless regrets, we should say encouragingly, 'I can do better'!

Man in evolution is subject to this iron law of karma. The smallest happening caused in the past will show its results in the future. Our karma of today is our free will of the past and free will of today is shaping the future in this and the next life.

Through every action, karma, the law of the universe, builds for certain results. This is the most exalted law. When we see it working in our daily life, when we understand it, it will help us take the biggest step towards self-realisation. Then we shall be able to accept every happening in our life as karma. If, in careless driving, we injure an innocent person and cripple him for life, is it not just that we will be reborn with a deformity? Once we really and truly understand this we are not able to hurt people any more.

As action always brings reaction, some people reason that no action would be the solution. Karma is not only physical action, it includes thinking and feeling, there is never a moment of inactivity in man's life. We should enjoy life fully, always exploring new avenues of knowledge while at the same time striving for peace of mind and kindness to every living being.

With every thought, with every action, we build a new karma, good or bad, depending entirely on the pureness of motive and action. Our reaction to what karma brings us today is already shaping new karma. It is quite unimportant what people say or do to us, as not a hair can be touched on our head without the will of God — it is our reaction which counts. Our reaction to any happening in our life will shape our future life. It is all so absolutely just that it needs the human nature to revolt against it!

One type of karma acts like a boomerang; the thrower is hit by his own thrust. As he directs his harmful action against another person it will rebound to him sooner or later, either in this or his subsequent life. Another kind of karma may manifest organically; a weak stomach in this life may be the direct consequence of uncontrollable gluttony in a previous existence. Yet another of the countless types of karma is symbolic, a lot of bloodshed in an earlier life having resulted in anaemia in this incarnation.

All pains and all limitations have an educational purpose. Deformities and other afflictions are of moral origin and all man's agonies are lessons in a long-term school for wisdom and perfection. All suffering has a cause and effect relationship, even if the cause came from a previous life and is, therefore, unknown to us. It is the law of compensation; what-so-ever a man soweth, that shall he also reap. Newton's third law of motion, namely, that every action has its reaction, which is equal and opposite, applies as much to the law of morals as to that of physics.

Heaven and Hell have to be known by the individual before he can discriminate between them. As long as emotions have not been mastered, reincarnation has to recur until man has overcome all shortcomings, until he has reached the state of perfect man. Reincarnation means evolution; the evolution of man through many life times lived on earth as a man or a woman, as a pauper or a king, belonging to one colour or another, until, finally, the being has reached the state of perfection.

Every new life in the chain of incarnations will result in a different personality. Each personality of a soul is a separate experience, in no way related to the other earlier experiences of the soul, except by common inclusion in the total of that being. Only when a lesson is perfectly understood can we go ahead and turn over a new page in the book of learning.

Unfoldment and experience are for ever linked together. As soon as we have understood the lesson of a certain experience, the explanation on the conscious level is achieved. The successful experience brings the previously unsolved emotional problem out of the dark into the light. There is an unending reorganisation and reorientation; with each lesson learned another aspect of life has to be faced. The more alert and conscious we are, the easier the constant change. Only when full consciousness is established can stability be achieved. That would be the state of perfect man, the state of immortality, man freed from the need to incarnate, free to choose if he is to work on earth or in the universe.

A rhythm that defies all sound
flows through the dark deep husk of soul
and stirs the sleeping glow of forgotten life.
So the cube melts in the sea,
and the sea, caught by the sun
— a tear drying on warm skin —
lifts into the sky to rise on waves
to the heart of its love
where the swan of eternity sings
in its career across the blue sky
of infinity.

M.B.

The more a human being evolves, the more he will use his emotions in a positive way. A quick tempered person will always be quick in changing emotions, but he will be in control of it and be the master of any situation. The greater his control over his emotions the more will his talents develop. There will first be a very strong and marked individualisation with definite talents. Genius is he who is born with one or more outstanding qualities. In the beginning the pressure of these talents may occasionally irritate and even un-balance the genius as we can frequently see in the tempestuous outbursts of some famous great men. The higher the advancement, the more numerous the capacities, the more even tempered and balanced the human being will be.

The solar system offers a cycle of experience for the evolving soul. It has seven dimensions corresponding to the seven principles of man — the seven planes, each having different conditions and dimensions. The earth is the third dimension and it is a kind of laboratory for the whole solar system, because on our earth free will is much stronger than on other planets. On the other planets, or dimensions, some measure of control is kept over the soul to see that it learns the proper lessons. The control is usually exercised by the soul itself, provided it has evolved sufficiently, because once the physical body of the earth dimension has been left behind and the consciousness of that life has been absorbed into the subconscious, the separation between the two is lifted.

The subconscious is the record of all the different lives of the soul, in this system as well as in the other systems out amongst the stars. It is the record we think of as being kept by the recording angels. In this Akashic Record is the story of what we do with our soul — that portion of God that is given to us for Life Eternal with the gift of individuality, or separate existence from God. Our aim is to perfect our individuality so that it is like the spirit and so that the two can merge and then, merged, return to God on the end of this Evolution.

Pre-birth memories exist deep in the subconscious, deeper than is usually reached by psychotherapy. The unconscious mind is more easily accessible to other unconscious minds than to the conscious mind. We have this experience quite frequently with kindred souls; before we express a thought, they have already picked it up and pronounce it, or we say it spontaneously together.

5

Self and Self-Image

In casual conversation the terms 'individuality' and 'personality' are often confused; they are considered to be synonymous and few people are really aware of the profound differences which make them two very distinct concepts.

Every human being has a basic structure and from the very beginning there is a certain inclination. This pre-dominance rules the life of each being. This really is the individual; it is the emotional part of man, his soul, and decides his approach to problems and decisions.

When a child is born he brings with him race-memory, the family traits of the parents, his own special make-up and the 'I am consciousness'; in one word, his individuality or, the basic structure of every newly born, his soul. It is the sum total of the positive experiences of all previous lives. It will be the reason for his inclinations and will affect his outlook on life and the way he makes decisions. The individuality is the true self — the innermost core — the essence of a being.

Man, therefore, is never born the same twice; he adds more wisdom through each new life, thus following the law of evolution. Every atom contains the impulse to reach for a higher form of life. It is that ever present impulse which urges on all living beings until, at last, fulfilment is achieved.

Compared with the immortal individuality, personality is only of this world and is mortal. A soul can never have the same personality twice because it has to be built anew in each incarnation. The building of the personality starts immediately after birth as it is the result of the impressions of the environment.

Man and his individuality — the inner-self — shows how far he has progressed on his way towards reunion with the immortal spark within him.

The personality — self-image — on the other hand is the playball of environment. It is, in other words, wide open to the influences of the circumstances and conditions into which we are born. Personality manifested by the behavioural manners and ways of each person and its development is subject to continuous effort. Conscious, vital efforts in particular determine new attitudes, which, when deeply established as a habit, add to the basic individuality in preparation for the next incarnation.

The personality is the superficial side of a being. Personalities are acquired after birth, being the direct result of environment, continent, country, colour, race, religion, upbringing and education, all of which play a certain role; very often more negative than anything else, because children have to fit into an established mould rather than the mould being adjusted to each child. The personality then is the least real part of a human being, but it frequently overgrows the individuality and overshadows the essence.

The individuality is the deepest core of our being, concealing the most profound emotions. All of these we tend to keep hidden, preferring to appear to the world wearing a mask, our personality. So you see, the personality is the least real part of a human being, but it is inclined to obliterate the soul or the individuality.

A well-balanced human being is the direct result of harmony between his 'individuality' and 'personality' and it is to achieve this that modern psychology, yoga and the now abundant psycho-scientific literature come to our aid. As will be pointed out in our explanation of yoga relaxation, everything is interdependent; so the relatively recent science of the self-image, in connection with psycho-cybernetics, also comes into our field of study.

What is this so-called self-image? It is my idea of what sort of a person I am and I have built this picture on my past successes, failures, emotions, joys, fears, my reactions to people and people's reaction to me, my environment, circumstances and on childhood experiences. From all these I have created a biased picture, or an image, of what

I think I am; and in doing so I have built up for myself a personality, which is, more likely than not, a mask. But to me it is a true picture and I have impressed it upon my subconscious.

All my actions, emotions and manners, but most importantly, my abilities, are developed in direct relation to the image I have built up of myself. If, for example, I believe myself to be completely hopeless with figures, I will indeed make a failure of everything that I am asked to do in this connection, purely because my 'hopelessness' stems, on examination, from the fact that in my early school years an impatient teacher made the remark that I was hopeless with figures.

In other words, self-image sets the boundaries of our abilities, limits us, ties our hands, and handcuffs us to failure for life. Until a little while ago it was considered that we were as we were and this was just bad luck and could not be helped.

Recent discoveries in the fields of science and psychology have disproved this theory of fatalism and it has been established that the self-image is very much susceptible to change and that the somewhat over-used phrase, 'turning failure into success', is applicable to anyone who wishes to apply it.

We must deviate for a moment to look at those recent scientific events which have led psychologists to their findings. It all happened during the Second World War and in the years immediately following. Remarkable observations were made in connection with work done on electronic devices, such as computers, guided missiles, torpedoes and the spacecraft of today. They were, and are, so constructed as to be goal-orientated mechanisms, i.e. once launched and set for their target, this is the only thing they aim to reach. They carry a sense device, such as radar, which, should they stray from course, will register this fact through a feed-back system, which will then automatically right the mechanism back to its correct course, steering it to the appointed target. The word 'cybernetics' comes from the Greek and means, literally, 'steersman'.

While Professor Norbert Wiener was working on these goal-orientated mechanisms to perfect them, he came to the conclusion that something analogous is happening in the human brain and that man is also so constructed as to hold within himself a success-striving, goal-minded mechanism, namely the subconscious, which is the servo-mechanism and which is directed by the conscious mind through the brain and nervous system. And so, after much research, technology and physics and modern psychology wedded themselves into what is known today as psycho-cybernetics.

By no means does this still new off-shoot of psychology maintain that man is a servo-mechanism. It does prove, however, that he has such a built-in mechanism which he can use for success as well as for failure. This is no different from what those of you who study esotericism have come to know in connection with thought-dynamics; the thought you send out will come back to you in kind. If you think joyously you will be surrounded by joy, if you think gloom, gloom will become yours, if you think health and love, they will be yours in time. If you think success, success will come to meet you and, likewise, if you think negatively and along lines of failure, these will be your target.

Even your body, as such, is success-striving. If one organ becomes deficient another will immediately strive to make compensation in one form or another. A cut, damaging tissues, will instantly strive to right itself through the calling into play of such agents in our physiological make-up as are required to effect healing. And again, we find something similar in a blind person who will usually be compensated for the loss of eyesight by developing other faculties to a more pronounced degree than someone with normal sight. So you see, man is fundamentally and basically goal-orientated.

Looking at it from an even higher viewpoint, it should be seen that each incarnation is part of the 'off-course adjustment', the successful steering, via trial and error, to man's final target — union with the Absolute. We can purposefully try to speed up this process with the various methods offered us by Yoga, such as relaxation, concentration, meditation and mind control in general.

Our servo-mechanism, the brain and the nervous-system, is not unlike a computer. No computer has quite the complexity of the human brain and it would be a long while, if ever, before this could be technologically achieved. To do this, to prepare and produce the right answer, we have to feed the mechanism with the right data; if we give it wrong information to work with it will necessarily give back the wrong answer. Likewise, if we hope to achieve success in our lives, in no matter which direction, we too must give our thought processing servo-mechanism the right thought food. Our self-image sets the limits to the boundaries of our abilities and achievements. If our self-image is such as to make us believe of ourselves that we are incompetent at drawing or at jumping, to take very simple examples, then that is what we are. This we will remain for the rest of our lives, unless we change our self-image, and, through it, enlarge and extend the limits of our abilities. Man is limitless; only wrong thought patterns place obstacles and barriers in his way and hinder his ascent.

By changing our self-image we change our whole personality and by consciously adopting new habit patterns we impress these on our subconscious and impregnate them with our individuality.

How then do we go about implementing this change? What is the method? Obviously, before we can effect any such change we must know what we want to change; we must consciously want to rid ourselves of old inhibitions. We must practice self-awareness to help us understand those actions and reactions in our make-up which hinder our progress.

Inhibitions and repressed experiences which have gone underground in our subconscious act as a hindrance to our intelligence. They prevent individuality and personality from working in union. Before we can achieve a new habit pattern we must clear out this old residue of the past. The transcendental quality of Progressive Yoga Relaxation will be of great help.

As explained, to produce the right answer, we have to feed our goal-orientated mechanism the right ideas.

Since earliest childhood we have confused the real with the unreal and we have replaced the truth with wishful thinking. When things become difficult, in self-pity, we escape in daydreams, feeding illusions to the subconscious till they seem real. At various stages of our life some of these fantasies have been shattered leaving us disappointed and depressed. If it is one of our main illusions that has been destroyed, we hate the whole world, including ourselves, and in an extreme case this leads to suicide.

Even level headed and mature people cherish a few illusions and are most unwilling to dismiss them. There are many, but I will only mention a few, the more commonplace ones.

Do you expect marriage to be: 'and they lived happily ever after'? Marriage is give and take, the most wonderful union between a man and a woman, but also the most demanding and most difficult. Love can never be taken for granted, it needs constant adjustment and must be handled like the most fragile, precious jewel.

Can you face growing older, being less attractive, less agile with no one paying any attention to you? Some women expect eternal youth, and most men everlasting virility.

Do you still dream of some far-away island — a heaven on earth, where everyone is beautiful, where there is only love, joyful living and happiness, where there is no competition, no work, only play?

In changing your self-image from fantasy to reality you have to destroy all the illusions of your dreams. You must realise you created this illusion and you are therefore the reason for your disillusions. Your disappointments are self-produced.

These illusions are part of the hypocrisy of our society. From earliest childhood, we are fed, daily, this diet of hypocrisy; through books, newspapers, radio, television, films. It is very frustrating and tedious to separate fantasy from truth, but it is the way to maturity, contentment and happiness.

As a rule, young people gain faster results than older ones who have to rid themselves of life-long habits and repressions. The most disciplined person finds it the hardest to go very deep, therefore they should not be discouraged, they must just persevere until they have results.

Having discarded old habits, one has to be most vigilant to make sure that they do not sneak back. As we are creatures of habit, we have to beware of these old patterns.

Once we have done so, we have next to create and experience the new characteristic which is to replace the old one; we have to create a new thought-habit pattern and impress it on the grey matter of our brain, the storehouse of our memory. If, in thought or deed, we impress the subconscious with success, we will identify ourselves, even more, with success.

To develop a realistic self-image we have to use our creative mechanism. Our imagination must come into play to bring about success in achieving our target. To do this we must first create a mental picture and experience it in our imagination — act it out in our imagination as if it were a live experience, not just a pictured one. A strong and vivid conscious visualization is as effective on our subconscious as an actual life experience.

Method:

1   Establish your target.
2   Relax.
3   Build up your target-image with absolute concentration, acting it out in your mind.
4   Do this for a period of twenty-one days, always keeping the same time.
5   When experienced to the full, detach your image, as it were, from its base and pass it to your subconscious.

It is important not to antagonise and confuse your servomechanism by living, during the day, in an opposite manner to the new image you have passed on to it.

Anxiety and Fear

Among the destructive forces which hinder our advancement in consciousness are lack of faith, and any kind of anxiety, fear, phobia, neurosis, or trauma.

In our time, the late 20th century, there is more fear than there has ever been before. Most evil arises from fear. Fear is the root from which fear grows. Only the real mystic is free from fear because of the contact he has with his soul. Such a state of inner peace of mind can be reached after conscious searching and work on one's self, and also through Progressive Yoga Relaxation and meditation. It is possible for everyone who makes the effort.

Mr. S. had an aversion to porridge. He explained that until now it had not bothered him, in fact he had forgotten all about it. However, now it was different, because of his promotion a year ago he had to travel continuously, and could not avoid coming across the smell of it, and it upset him for the whole day. He experienced a sort of deep down unease; it affected his relationship with people and made him rather unsure of himself. He had tried to play more golf, took a very vigorous course in weight-lifting and his doctor had even sent him to a psychiatrist to no avail, so a friend suggested Progressive Yoga Relaxation.

Whenever Mr. S. was in Melbourne he came to a relaxation class. He progressed quite well, and was able to cope better, but still had his aversion. I had insisted that he must not avoid it through having breakfast in his room or missing breakfast altogether. The worst thing to do is to avoid a phobia, as it is self-winding.

Finally, through his perseverance with Progressive Yoga Relaxation exercises and his determination not to avoid his aversion, Mr. S. came face to face with his problem. He was able to spring the lock of his memory where, hidden away deep in his subconscious, there lay the childhood experience that was the root of his phobia.

Thus it came to a head. As a very small child, he was sitting with his great-grandmother on the hearth, and she was feeding him porridge. He was holding a little wooden horse in his hand waving it about, he threw it, unintentionally, into the coal fire. Before the great-granny could prevent him, he reached for it and burned his hand badly. The pain made him vomit and from then on he did not want porridge and if forced to take it, he vomited and was sick for the rest of the day.

We each have some kind of subconscious fear which permeates our life and influences everything we do. Every average person has at least one, if only very small, phobia. This is simply a dread or uncontrollable fear. It may be of a morbid character, or merely a fear of some object or situation. You realise that your fear is utterly ridiculous, but you feel powerless to do anything about it. You may have tried to ignore it only to find that this does not work. It still has the power to tie your stomach in knots. It can not be reached through the conscious mind as it is seated in the subconscious.

One person is afraid of his marriage partner, another fears the dark, some fear the drive of their sexual urges, others that they won't have enough money. Some fear the opinion of their neighbours. Birds can be the reason for fear, or mice, or cats. But worst of all is the fear of the unknown which grips the heart with an iron hand, leaving us gasping for air, covered in cold sweat and utterly exhausted. Behind this dark, undefined fear lurks the greatest of all fears — the fear of death.

In primitive races fears are even stronger than with civilised people and the breaking of taboos often leads to death, such as happens after 'the pointing of the bone' by the Australian Aborigines.

Each personality differs, but people may be roughly divided into categories according to the way they solve their conflicts.

The Immature: This first kind merely capitulates to primitive desires. People in this class may not be nervous, but they are not happy either. The voice of the conscience is hard to drown, even when it is not strong enough to control our conduct. But happily for us when we desert the ways of ethical conduct our conscience often succeeds in making us miserable. The immoral person has, as yet, not come to recognise the possibility of a self-directed life; he simply disregards the collective wisdom of our society and gives the victory to those primitive forces which try to keep man back on his old level. We cannot ignore the ethical standards by which man lives, and still be happy.

The Mature: These people decide their conflicts in a way which satisfies both themselves and society. They give the victory to higher trends and at the same time make a lasting peace by winning over the energies of the undesirable impulses. By sublimating them they divert the threatening forces to useful work, channelling them into real life and using the power to make the world's wheels go around. Their love force, unhampered by childish habits, is free to give itself to mature adult relationships or to express itself symbolically in socially helpful ways.

The Neurotic: In this third group we find people who, as yet, have not finished the fight. These are the ones with nerves; the people in whom conflict is always present because both sides, the primitive and the guided ways, are equally strong. The victory goes to neither side; the tug of war — the unending struggle — continues. Since the energy of the nervous person is divided between the effort to repress and the effort to gain expression, there is little strength left for the external world, for contact with mankind. There is plenty of energy wasted on emotion, fantasy or useless acts symbolising the struggle.

The neurotic type of person is a normal person — only more so! Everything about him is overdone. His impulses are the same as those of every other person, his complexes are the same kind of complexes, only more intense. He is, so to speak, larger than life. He may be only slightly exaggerated, showing merely a little character weakness, or he may be so intensified that everything is out of focus. In that case, he makes life miserable for himself and for everybody around him. It is quantity not quality that ails him. He has too much of everything, for he differs from his neighbour, not in kind, but in degree. Most of himself is repressed and the larger part of him is fixed in a childish mould.

On the physical level we are able to survive because our body has practically unlimited restorative power. Take, for example, a broken leg, it will heal and be stronger than ever without any exterior help. What the doctor does is to make sure that the fractured pieces knit in the right way, but the healing process, as such, lies entirely in the nature of each patient. It is the same with a cold or with a simple cut. The body continues to live, not by complete avoidance of danger, but by a constant righting of what goes wrong. Every second of our life there is that adjustment and renewal taking place, hence any abnormal failure of the body to achieve self-healing is a symptom to be taken seriously; it is a warning of some impaired functioning of the organism.

Most people never give a thought to the body's wonderful recuperative power. Only when it does not function do they worry, and go to the doctor.

On the emotional level these same recuperative powers apply, and are even more important. The personality structure, like the body, lives in a world where hurtful things happen. The mental and emotional health is maintained, not by avoiding injury, but by recuperating from injury, from all the wounds our surroundings inflict on our soul.

Mrs. F. was in her early thirties, but hardly a day passed that she did not burst into tears. She just could not cope with the increasing duties of being the wife of a chief executive and with the ever-increasing demands of four children. She had always blushed easily and the slightest exertion made her hot and sticky. Through Progressive Yoga Relaxation she came to re-live a forgotten episode of her early childhood:

When her grandmother went to live with them she had to share her room with her. She was used to sleeping with an open window, but now the window was closed. She hated the smell of the room, but she hated even more, because she was rather reserved and shy, the old lady's constant kissing and cuddling. This brought about punishment from her mother.

Life was never the same again. The pattern was so set that it did not alter even after the grandmother's death, so she never regained a close relationship with her mother. In fact, she still feared and resented her till this experience became clear to her through relaxation.

It was all so clear and she now can understand her mother and, at last, communicate with her. The blushing and perspiration have gone. She feels a different person and enjoys her interesting life.

Our recuperative powers enable us to become involved in the positive, dangerous business of living. If healing fails us, ordinary happenings can then prove overwhelming. The slightest injury, whether inflicted on a finger or on the ego, becomes a major problem. If a wound, be it physical or emotional, does not heal, it shows a state of ill-being which goes much further than the area of the wound.

The healthy person is resilient, has elasticity. This does not mean he does not feel hurt, but he recovers quickly. Small hurts will induce slight reactions; even major disappointments and griefs are accommodated, and taken as a lesson from life, and the healing leaves no marks.

To hold grudges or to hug a sense of humiliation for a prolonged period of time, are sure signs of maladjustment. Such a person comes to a psychological halt, unaware that life must go on.

Be sure not to confuse prompt recuperative power with heartlessness. Coldness can well be the end product of many hurts and is, in itself, a wrong way of protection. You must be able to take risks in life and enjoy it, unafraid of being hurt.

Some people tend to make an asset of their shortcomings and handicaps, unconsciously appealing to the pity of their fellow men.

Under no circumstances must we suppress emotions, natural or unnatural. They must be understood, sublimated and lifted on to a creative level. Suppressed feelings cause emotional habit patterns that inhibit our brain, nerves and organs.

Every human being has vast reservoirs of energy waiting to be used. When our efforts are fired by the energy of right emotions, the flow of abundant force astonishes us. But our strength fails us frequently because our energy is locked up by negative emotions and fear. With understanding we can lead this basic flow of energy into music, art, technical invention, business, sport or any other creative activity.

Repression of an emotion before it has reached the surface will produce harmful effects and the repressed energy will result in painful emotional habit patterns which we fail to understand. This causes more unhappiness and the start of a vicious circle. It is not the emotion, no matter how primitive, but the suppression, with the evil association we attach to it, that causes all the trouble.

We all know that the body reacts automatically to our thoughts. Think of a favourite dish and the mouth waters. Some people become very stimulated by suggestive talking about sex. Blushing is another example of such a reaction. Any strong emotion is registered in the part of the brain called the hypothalamus. This part immediately sends signals all over the body; we breathe deeper to fill the lungs with oxygen, the heart speeds up to rush the oxygen-charged blood all over the body, but especially to the muscles. At the same time hormones are poured into the blood-stream and carried as a booster to the nervous system. In a second the whole body is in excited anticipation of danger or pleasure.

How exactly does this state come about? The hypothalamus, that part of the brain which is in control of all the instinctive, primitive reactions like hunger, sex, anger, fear, jealousy and so on, is connected through a kind of stalk with the pituitary gland. This wonderful small gland, the size of an ordinary small marble, located about one and a half inches deep, straight in between the eyebrows at the base of the brain, was already known by ancient Greek philosophers, as well as in our own time, for its production of some growth hormones.

But only in recent years was it found that the front lobe triggers off the making of sex hormones, through releasing certain chemicals into the bloodstream. It also governs the thyroid, which in turn, controls the whole metabolism. Another of its chemical secretions helps the suprarenal gland to regulate its hormonal output. The middle and back lobes of the pituitary stimulate the kidneys, affect the contraction of the uterus and regulate the blood pressure.

You will also recall the great importance of your lungs; amongst their many functions they eliminate two pounds of waste matter a day, which is equivalent to that thrown off by the bowels and kidneys. Not only does proper breathing eliminate waste but it has a profound effect on our emotional nature. Only when we breathe properly will we be ready to review our mental make-up, including all those emotional reactions and repressed painful memories going as far back as the first months.

Man, the highest being on this earth, must consciously do everything in his power to improve himself and go ahead in evolution. But for as long as he still represses every emotion not approved of by society, his progress will be extremely slow. In science, practically nothing can stop him, but his ethical advancement depends entirely on his emotional maturity. Man has to learn to face this primitive inheritance. He has to make peace with his instincts and instead of suppressing them, use them fully to his advantage. There is no greater force than the emotional drive. Because the elementary force of instinct is so powerful, people are afraid and ashamed of it. This fear and shame has to be overcome completely, not by making coarse jokes, but through an understanding of how the elementary instincts function. Unashamed, but without exhibitionism, we must understand these forces and use them for higher purposes. Man has no way of producing high-power energy other than through his emotions. It does not really matter how these forces come about, the important thing is to use them.

This does not mean that man has to become an introvert, plunged into self-analysis. No, he just has to accept his sexual drives as well as his destructive tendencies. Actually there is no emotion which has not to do with either self-preservation or procreation; without these all-powerful, ruthless instincts man could not have survived. Physically he is much too poorly equipped to have survived as a meek, gentle being. He needed every little bit of his aggressiveness to survive and he still needs it as much as ever, but in a sublimated form. He has to lift these primordial emotions from the instinctive level to the intellectual, or better still, the spirit-mind level. Then progress can accelerate and man will become more humane. This has to come about during the next decades, as the Aquarian time falls into a double cycle giving even greater importance to it and this is why our time will produce profound and unfathomable impact on the future.

Belief is unconditioned faith in the absolute power of God; it is a vibration and the same when an evolved being contacts the Absolute as when a primitive believes in the absolute power of a little statue. It is the same vibration and the results are the same. It is the greatest power in the Universe and with it mountains can be moved.

Faith is in the subjective mind and superstition is very often faith in the wrong things. If your faith is purely in the conscious mind, then it is an opinion. Only if an idea is accepted by your subconscious will it change your life. It is not an exaggeration to say that every human being is hypnotised or brain-washed to some extent, either by ideas he has uncritically accepted from others or ideas he has repeated to himself or statements from newspapers, advertisements, radio and television. This is how political and social ideas are implanted in the subjective mind.

Man today, is brainwashed by fear of the future and the consequences of interference with the ecology. He lives in dread of the effects of pollution and over-population; some are negative about the outer-space programme. Not only can we cope and find solutions to these problems (which, after all, are man-made) with our advanced scientific knowledge, but we can improve on and make this a lovelier world than it ever was. The good old days are a myth. They were only good for an extremely privileged few; a strike to reduce a sixty-three hour week was unsuccessful even in 1912! Sanitation was apalling. There was no refrigeration, causing a very unbalanced diet. Apart from a few advanced countries, compulsory education came only in the twenties. Social welfare was non-existent; there was only charity. Since there were no remedies for most of the contagious diseases, survival depended on the individual's constitution. Housekeeping was tedious and travelling hard and difficult. We should realize that we have never had it so good!

There is no difference between the skilled hypnotist and the methods of brainwashing just mentioned. The strongest man can be hypnotised so that he cannot lift a needle, and he can also be hypnotised into lifting much more than his usual capacity without ill-effect. It is really quite difficult not to assume that the hypnotist has magical power when you witness a good, genuine demonstration — the stutterer makes a fluent and wonderful speech, someone who usually plays the piano rather badly, plays it with skill and yet another, who maintains he cannot draw, makes a better than average portrait. But these performances have nothing to do with the hypnotist; all he did was to free the subjects of their wrong beliefs and inhibitions.

Under her affable manners Mrs. N. was hiding a profound and deep mistrust of people and a great inner loneliness. When she began Progressive Yoga Relaxation classes it took her longer than the average person to settle into the routine of the place and only after many courses did she finally reach below the surface to expose the terrifying experience that had given rise to her adult problems.

I was the youngest child in the family, with three brothers. When I was about two years old, our nanny was washing my hair when bathing me and when the soap got into my eyes, I screamed. Nanny became most annoyed. As her angry face came very near, I became frightened and screamed louder. She covered my face with one hand and with the other pushed me under the water. I was petrified and thought she would kill me, I struggled wildly, thrashing with my arms and legs, finally she let me sit up; I was completely breathless. At that moment my beloved mother entered the bathroom and having regained my breath, I howled at the top of my voice, expecting compassion from my mother. Nanny complained to mother about my ill-temper and said that the three boys, together, had not been half the trouble I was. My mother was angry and scolded me; and she left without a kind word and Nanny triumphantly shook me'.

Mrs. N. realises now that she never really overcame the shock of that terrifying moment. Having faced the cause of it all she now finds it much easier to reach and enjoy people and her whole life is more satisfying.

Most people have some kind of inferiority complex. It does not originate from facts or experiences, but from our wrong evaluation of experiences and our mistaken conclusions regarding facts. If you are an inferior driver, that does not make you an inferior person. The feeling of inferiority comes about for just one reason; comparing yourself with others. If you do not reach the standard of the other person you feel inferior, but you forget that you have qualities the other does not have. You are an individual, and as different in your mental make-up as you are in your physical constitution, so do not make comparisons.

Inferiority and superiority are the reverse sides of the same coin. You are not inferior, you are not superior; you are you. There really does not exist such a thing as the average or common man. You, as a personality, are not in competition with any other personality, simply because there is not another person on the face of the earth like you.

Most of you will want to try out all recommendations made in this book. Some of you will believe absolutely and follow them full of confidence and get marvellous results. Some will start well, but, after a few days, their doubtful nature will come to the fore and destroy all the progress achieved till now, and they will have to begin all over again. As soon as you doubt something you rub out your blueprint in the Universal Mind. Some will be doubtful from the beginning and say 'I may try'. Faith is absolute. Doubt is fear of failure and is fatal. Hope, wondering and questioning are not positive enough; they already contain the element of failure.

There is a story of a yogi who met Cholera on the way to Calcutta. The yogi enquired where it was going. 'To Calcutta', answered the Cholera, 'to slay ten thousand' — and departed. The yogi, unafraid of the plague, continued and finally arrived at the city, where he heard that a hundred thousand had died. Later on the two travellers met again, and the yogi asked the Cholera why he had lied to him. 'Oh no, I have not lied to you', replied the Cholera, 'I slew only ten thousand, the rest died of fear!'

This morning
Driving to town
The hot wind
Whirled yellow leaves
Across the intersection

In a flash
Complacent summer
Endless no more —
Like the first grey hair
Like wrinkles in morning mirrors
Reminders of time
A cold feeling of urgency.

                    B.M.

Breath is Life

Breathing is such an automatic function of the body that it is taken for granted by most of us. Very few give it a second thought, wonder what it is, or why and how we breathe, not to mention the general lack of awareness of the tremendous importance and far-reaching effects of this particular function of the body. Breathing is not a function on its own, it is connected with our entire well-being. Now that our way of life has become so motorised, that we scarcely ever walk, we have lost the art of deep breathing. It is quite staggering to realise just how few people breathe correctly.

The element air symbolises the law of breath, of life itself. The law is that we must give out as much as we have received or we cannot take in a full amount again. If we continue to give out and take in, in short measure, our lungs will cease to act properly and will become atrophied or diseased. You cannot get around it, if you abuse this law you will suffer, this is what is wrong with the world today and all International Conferences, and Peace Treaties on earth will be of no avail until we respect and practise this law.

Through the abuse of this law of give and take, fear has entered into our lives — fear that our possessions will be taken away from us; fear that we cannot keep what we have; fear that our enemy will invade us; fear that we might lose our job because of mental inefficiency; fear that we shall not have enough to eat. Do we not even hold our breath when we are afraid and does it not paralyse every function of our bodies? If, when we are afraid, we take seven long deep breaths, and breathe out in a very controlled and slow manner, with the exhaling taking rather longer than the inhaling — fear will vanish, because breath is courage.

When you are calm and peaceful, your breath is slow and even, with a pause of a few seconds before inhaling. When you are angry or agitated it is quick and uneven without an interval. When you control your breath, you are master of your mental and emotional state.

When I sat opposite the young pregnant woman my heart went out to her. She was breathing laboriously and her halting speech was constantly interrupted by gasping for air.

Her doctor, supported by her husband, thought it necessary to interrupt her pregnancy.

She wanted the baby and was willing to do anything to improve her breathing and overcome her fear. Her asthma dated from earliest childhood, in fact she could not remember a time without it and she had had all kinds of unsuccessful treatments over the years till at last she had resigned herself. Now she had only three weeks till her hospital booking and she was determined to have her baby.

She came every day for special pranayama and Progressive Yoga Relaxation. Her recovery was spectacular. It was one of those strange cases where nothing much happens, just a bit of anxiety and a bit of crying. Her husband was thrilled and her doctor was amazed and put it down to will power.

After her healthy boy was born she had a mild reoccurrence of asthma, which was overcome by a few sessions. They have three children now and after each birth she comes for a while.

I would like her to continue till she has a very strong reaction, but she just cannot find the time.

Breath is life, and life is rhythm. Without breathing there could be no life on earth. Man, the higher and lower animals, plant life, all depend on air for existence. Breathing is the most important of the bodily functions, all else being dependent on it. Man can go without food for days, or even weeks, but in order to survive he can only go without breath for a few minutes.

The moment a new-born babe leaves its mother's womb it inhales a first deep breath and then exhales with its first cry and — it lives! By taking this first breath — by commencing the alternating flow of inhalation and exhalation — the new body tunes into the rhythm of life with its positive and negative phases and stays in it until the moment of death when the last exhalation leaves the body.

If the intake of breath is the absolute pre-requisite for life, one would presume that man should be able to exercise the act of breathing with perfection. Unfortunately, this is not so. While plants and animals follow the dictates of nature, and while primitive man did so in his natural habitat, living in the open air and relying on hunting and fishing for sustenance, man in the 20th Century has almost completely forgotten how to breathe fully and correctly.

Those who work out of doors are somewhat less affected, but the millions who sit or stand, day in, day out, in offices, shops and factories, no longer know how to use their lungs effectively. Illness and disease, as well as an enormous amount of emotional imbalance, is the result.

Without going into too much anatomical detail, we should try to have at least some idea of the respiratory system, its mechanics and functions.

That the lungs are the main mechanism is common knowledge, but generally speaking little else is known. Air passages lead to the two lungs, these air passages start with the nose and, of course, the mouth. The nose is equipped with a filter system of fine hairs and mucous membranes which are of importance for cleansing and adjusting the air to the body temperature. It is for this reason that nasal breathing is so strongly advocated, mouth breathing being more or less taboo because the mouth lacks all the preventative equipment of the nose. Next in the air passages comes the pharynx, the larynx and the windpipe or trachea which develops into a larger air-tube branching out into two sets of tubes leading to the lungs; these tubes are known as the bronchials. The two lungs are separated by the mediastinum and the heart. The lungs themselves consist of a porous elastic-like tissue filled with blood vessels, capillaries and millions of air cells, the alveols. If the air cells of the lungs were spread over an unbroken area, end to end, they would cover 14,000 feet. The lungs themselves are covered by a delicate, but strong, plastic-like tissue known as the pleural sac which, with its fluid secretion, contributes to the smoothly gliding action of breathing. Please realise and understand that these details are very fundamental, but adequate for the immediate purpose.

Similarly, let us briefly look at the system of blood circulation which is so utterly dependent on breath. The fresh blood starts its journey through the body from the left side of the heart through the arteries, bright red in colour, rich and vital, and returns, after a full circuit to the right portion of the heart through the veins, blueish, dark, filled with waste matter collected on its journey through the body. The right side now turns over this waste-filled blood to the fine capillaries in the lungs. As a fresh breath is inhaled and the oxygen in the air makes contact with the waste and poison-filled venous blood, a kind of combustion occurs. The blood absorbs the fresh oxygen and simultaneously releases the carbon dioxide generated by the waste and poisonous matter. Thus, purification of the blood takes place and the heart perpetuates the circulation with yet more vital and life-giving nourishment for the whole body.

The lungs and the heart are situated in the thoracic cavity which is the portion between the neck and the abdomen. Its boundaries are the spine, the ribs, the breast bone, and the diaphragm, a muscular partition between the thorax and abdomen. This portion, the thoracic cavity is better known to all of us as the chest. From the spine issue, protectively, twelve pairs of ribs; of these twelve pairs, the upper seven are called the true ribs because they are fastened to the breastbone. The others are false or floating ribs, the first three pairs are fastened to each other by cartilage, while the two remaining float free and so allow for greater elasticity.

The intercostal muscles and the diaphragm are responsible for moving the ribs. As the muscles cause the rib-cage to expand during inhalation, a vacuum is created and the required amount of air rushes in, and conversely, by the contracting action of the muscles the diaphragm moves back into place, a narrowing down of the ribs results and the air is pressed out. It is evident therefore that correct breathing depends to a large extent on the correct action of the muscles to enable maximum expansion and contraction of the lungs.

Now that you have a little more knowledge of the basic function of breathing and its close link with the blood circulation it will be clearer to you why so much stress is placed on correct and efficient breathing. The greater and more complete the intake of air and oxygen, the richer and healthier will be the blood feeding the entire body and the more thorough the cleansing process through the release of poisonous gases and waste material. The richly oxygenated blood will not only benefit your body physically, keep cells and tissues in perfect health, the organs well irrigated and tuned, your skin clear and fresh, but it brings immense benefits mentally.

Those who are able to breathe properly have an alert keen mind, think clearly, and are 'right on the ball'. (This is why in Hatha Yoga, so much emphasis is placed on breathing.) When breathing is not up to par, particularly in those who sit for hours at a desk, there is a tendency, after a while, to feel hazy, especially in the head. All functions appear to have slowed down and the person feels he would just like to curl up in a corner and go to sleep. The body objects instinctively and acts; your mouth opens for a heart-rending yawn, and your arms go up for a good stretch. Without being conscious of what you have done, you have made yourself breathe deeply, or as deeply as you are capable of, and replenished your oxygen-starved system.

What the lack of deep breathing does to your mind is quite obvious, but what is not so noticeable is the altering of your character. A person with faulty breathing becomes narrow-minded, and loses a lot of the wonderful qualities which makes an outstanding human being; qualities such as compassion, broad-mindedness, logical thinking, daring, speculation of the mind and so on.

There is an Eastern proverb which says: 'He who knows the art of breathing has the strength, wisdom, and courage of ten tigers.'

It is of importance, therefore, that we should introduce such replenishing actions conscientiously and regularly into our daily lives, particularly during our working hours. Weekend sport is excellent for those who actively participate. Be sure, if it is at all possible, to sleep with the windows wide open all the year round. On rising take three full breaths in front of the open window. It is always good to finish off your shower with the water completely cold; this most certainly ensures that you take at least a few deep breaths.

It is so simple to establish the habit of correct breathing in your everyday life, and several times during the day to take a few deep breaths. All of this will, in time, bring you great physical and mental benefits. Many debilities can be alleviated and in some cases eliminated altogether, such as respiratory troubles, colds, asthma, etc. The greater muscular activity through more intensive and proper breathing will gently massage the internal organs tuning up the entire metabolism.

We have discussed the parts of the anatomy involved, and some of the benefits to be enjoyed; now on to the practical: Breathing is a natural function, it is part of us and has to be easy and without force. The air must not be sucked in, the nose is only a channel, the air must flow in gently. Breathing is done in three parts — lower, middle, upper; or abdomen, thorax and highest chest.

In the first part the diaphragm moves down bringing the abdomen slightly out, through this a vacuum is created and the air streams in. (Wherever there is a vacuum on Earth, air automatically fills it without any effort on the part of the vacuum. The same applies to man, for whom all snivelling and sucking in of air is the wrong technique.) Secondly the ribs expand sideways taking in more air and, thirdly, the chest lifts slightly making space for even more air.

The most important part of each breath action is the abdominal; it takes in the most air, then comes the thorax and then the chest. All three phases should be used in every normal breath in that order. It is essential to keep each phase till the whole lungs are full, because, if the diaphragm is allowed to go up as the ribs are widened, the used air of the lower part of the lungs is filling the middle part of the lungs with the already used air giving a feeling of lack of air and frustration. Try it out and you will experience it. There should be an interval of about three seconds before the next inhaling. This technique is called Yogi-breathing.

If this breathing technique is contrary to your concept, observe a naked baby breathe. You will see a perfect example of diaphragm breathing. You may wonder what brings about the change from correct to incorrect breathing.

It comes about slowly in the small child through too much tension caused by shock and disturbance. Every toddler is frequently bombarded with — 'do not do that', 'do this' and so on. He unconsciously anticipates these commands, no matter how friendly they are expressed, they are orders and he protects himself in advance through tensing of the diaphragm. If this becomes a habit he uses his diaphragm insufficiently or in the reverse way and this produces shallow or wrong breathing.

In all the thousands of people to whom I taught breathing, the right technique was the exception and not the norm, with the exception of athletes, sportsmen and singers.

If correct breathing is accepted, and has become fully automatic, and is even up-kept in moments of great stress, it shows a well-adjusted, healthy being. A lot of people, trained to breathe correctly, reverse to the old habit when under strain, showing a latent, unsolved problem. They should continue with regular breathing exercises and Progressive Yoga Relaxation until there is no reversion even under the greatest stress.

Mrs. E. had such strong asthma that she could only sleep when under heavy sedation and during bad weather she needed daily injections. After a few weeks she did not require them any more. She also slept well and only in exceptionally humid weather did she have to take sedatives.

This was all she wanted. To avoid a reoccurrence I made her continue Progressive Yoga Relaxation for many weeks at home till she had the following experience:

I had started to wet my bed again after the divorce of my parents. Before leaving for boarding school Nanny tried unsuccessfully to cure me through severe punishments. The first day at the school I only thought of the night and how to avoid being laughed at. At last I found a solution; never to sleep at night in bed. I sat the whole night and prayed to the Holy Virgin and stayed awake, but I fell asleep in class and in chapel. This went on for a week or so till one night I fell asleep and woke up dry next morning. I was wonderfully relieved and took it as an answer from the Holy Mother. That day I had the first asthma attack and they reoccurred increasingly till I had it all the time plus very severe attacks.

Relaxation, pranayama and Hatha Yoga helped me and now I am completely free of asthma.

Before leaving the practical side of breathing, there is one other part worth cultivating. Not only do we breathe through the nose, but, to a lesser degree, through the pores of the skin. This very vital, oxygenating process takes place in the filigree network of the capillaries, which extend right into the skin tissues themselves. These capillaries, on a smaller scale, aid the work carried out by the blood vessels of the lungs. It is most important therefore, that the pores of the skin should be free to admit the flow of the air to reach these capillaries. The more the air has access to the skin surface the better. Even in winter we should try not to imprison the skin too much with heavy clothing and to spend at least some time each day entirely naked.

Before the daily bath or shower, it is good to brush vigorously the entire (dry) skin surface with a dry brush, to take out of the pores every last bit of matter which could obstruct the desired air-flow. Do not worry, a strong brushing will not in any way harm your skin. Touch it after the brushing and you will find it softer and smoother than before.

Esotericists believe that air contains a substance or principle from which stems all vitality — energy — life. This substance is called, 'Prana'. Prana is a Sanskrit word meaning life-force or vital-energy. It is the active principle in life. It is found in all forms of life from the most elementary mineral life to the highest form of animal life. It pervades everything, is in everything, it is the intangible force that maintains life in the Universe. If we think of Prana as being the active principle of what we call vitality, we will be able to form a much clearer idea of what an important part it plays in our lives — just as oxygen in the bloodstream is used up by the needs of the system.

We are constantly inhaling air charged with Prana. In ordinary breathing we absorb and extract a normal supply of Prana, but in controlled and regulated breathing greater supplies can be taken in and put to different uses. It can be absorbed into the system and can be stored in the nervous system as well as in the blood.

Breath can be used both inwardly and outwardly. Outwardly it is used to give additional benefits by exercising the body. Inwardly it is applied to create an appropriate inner atmosphere, conducive to mind control, concentration and meditation. We combine it in order to make a greater impact on the body or a special chosen part of it, through a mental command strengthened by breathing. We also use the external physical action to bring about an internal emotional reaction. For example a person trembling with excitement, and with a very fast pulse, can be calmed by inducing deep even breathing. Fear, or worry, or even suspicion can be alleviated and the reverse moods established. With practice you can achieve any condition or habit you wish in connection with self-improvement — all simply by correct breathing.

If you have a quality you feel requires improving — perhaps you are very impatient and this tends to distress you and annoy others — you can help and strengthen your decision for self-improvement through breathing exercises. Through an act of your conscious mind you create evenly this picture in your subconscious mind which will become fortified by Prana; it will grow clearer and stronger, and you will feel your patience increasing. You must then make use of every possible opportunity in everyday life to control impatience, and consciously supplant it with patience.

This method of self-improvement can be used on all short-comings. The more often you practice it, and the greater the regularity, the more effective will be the results.

Breathing Exercises

One of the biggest problems of the Royal Air Force during the Second World War was the loss of men and machines through battle fatigue of the pilots. What baffled the RAF most was the lack of pattern in breakdowns; some cracked up after a small number of flights, others doubled or tripled this statistic for no apparent reason and there were the few pilots who just did not get unduly affected by strain and never broke down.

Most people would consider this as normal — different personalities, different reactions. But in the case of the fighter pilots there was more to it. Pilots had to pass the most severe, precise, multifarious and vigorous tests. Nothing was left to chance as the pilots, as well as the machines, were irreplaceable. All the men had similar reactions to the tests and therefore basically a lot in common.

At last, near the end of the war the researchers found a very peculiar item. It was checked and re-checked, but it stood up to all tests. Those pilots who had the longest interval between exhaling and inhaling again were practically immune to stress. The shorter the interval the quicker the breakdown. This fact conforms with the yoga technique of breathing. This long interval (two to four seconds) is proof of presence of mind, even under the greatest strain.

There are countless variations of breathing exercises. To know a few of them so well that they are performed automatically, is all that is really needed. Only when your yogi-breathing is well established, practice the following exercises in the given sequence.

Start with five minutes practising extending to ten once you are proficient at it. As soon as you know the exercises use them consciously during mechanical work, in walking before going to sleep, in fact, wherever you can fit them in, till at last correct breathing is part of your life.

The measure of counting is your own pulse which means approximately a second for each count . . .

Various Breathing Exercises (Pranayama)

The skin is like a second set of lungs, like another pair of kidneys. For this reason it should be kept in a very good condition. Before the daily shower, the whole body should be brushed with a dry, hard brush. Use a rotating movement and work from the extremities towards the heart, including the face.

Even in the depth of winter the daily warm shower should finish with a cold shower, by turning off the hot tap and permitting the water to run cold — staying under it several minutes. Whilst under the shower remember to feel you are washing all negativeness away. To dry off, the healthiest way is to do active type exercise. A healthy, well functioning skin is aiding the lungs and the kidneys, helping to keep them in good condition.

Pore breathing: During breathing, concentrate only on the pores. In the beginning, feel it in one hand, or in the face, later on you will be able to feel it over the whole body.

Everything in the Universe vibrates and is part of the cosmic rhythmical law; high tide and low tide, summer and winter, day and night, to mention just a few of them.

The human body is also subject to the law of rhythm. Man can tune in by using his own heart beat as a count to his breathing.

Rhythmical breathing: Always be at ease before you start; sitting up straight with loose, relaxed shoulders.

Inhale counting six pulse beats.

Retain the breath for three pulse beats.

Exhale softly with closed mouth during six pulse beats.

Count three pulse beats before you start again.

Try to achieve a wonderful even flow, till the breathing happens alone, instinctively.

Calming breathing: To the count of seven, low and effortless abdominal breathing; also warming.

Waking up breathing: As soon as you are out of bed do seven of it.

Stand erect, feet slightly apart, hands in front on the thighs.

As you inhale, simultaneously rise on the tip of your toes and lift your arms high and as far back as possible.

Hold the position, and your breath, up to five pulse beats.

Let the body drop forward, completely relaxed, and at the same time exhale with an open mouth.

Invigorating breathing: Stand erect, arms hanging relaxed on the sides. Full Yogi-breathing, the consciousness is in the spine and the chin slightly towards the throat, eyes fixed on a point about two metres in front of the eye level. The weight of the body resting lightly on the foot balls, so that slight swinging is possible. As soon as there is a feeling of balance, after inhaling seven, hold the breath for five seconds and think: 'Breath is life, spirit, health'.

As you go ahead with this pranayama you can inhale longer and hold longer, but there should never be any strain.

Vitalising breathing: Sit upright, yet very relaxed. Think of life-force as a golden light and realise, without it there would be no life.

Consciously fill your lungs with life-force (seven pulse beats).

Retain your breath for seven beats and as you exhale imagine the golden life-force streaming from your lungs to your head.

Repeat three times.

The next three breaths are directed to the right arm, then to the left arm, then to the right leg and then to the left leg.

With time you will be able to vitalise your whole body in one breath, sending life-force from the lungs in all directions.

If holding the breath causes you the slightest discomfort, start with less and increase carefully. In breathing exercises strain must be avoided at all cost.

Lung fortification breathing: Lie on the ground, heels together, palms facing the floor.

Inhale, then press hands, feet and head strongly to the ground, and retaining the breath, hold the position. Let go during exhaling of seven. Three times.

Dynamic lung fortification breathing: Same as before but this time arch your body as much as possible during the holding of the breath (three times). Afterwards lie still and be conscious of the activation of the blood circulation in the lungs. This pranayama is best done in the garden or on the beach. In three weeks you will experience great improvement. Moderation and steadiness are the two important factors in breathing.

Simple Chakra breathing: Put right thumb on right nostril, middle finger and forefinger between the eyebrows, ring finger and little finger on the left nostril. Keep all fingers in place, then, as you inhale, lift your thumb only, so that you inhale through the right nostril (three seconds). Close the right nostril again and hold your breath for twelve seconds. Open the left nostril and exhale six seconds. Inhale left nostril, three seconds, close the nostril and hold your breath during twelve seconds, exhale right, six seconds. Repeat seven times. Once the technique is mastered you can use it to cure migraine; during the period, in which you hold your breath for twelve seconds, you imagine life-force sweeping backwards and forwards through your brain to activate the blood circulation in the brain and the skull, and, last, sweep it out of the head.

Peace breathing: Sitting in lotus position or on a chair, hands folded with forefingers outstretched and pointing towards the floor.

During three deep breaths concentrate strength between the eyebrows.

Next breath: Breathe in and send the concentrated strength from the forehead as a golden beam charged with peace and good-will into the Universe, or in a specific area which needs peace.

This golden beam of light can also be sent to a friend in need, but it has to be used altruistically in universal love, not in personal attachment.

Before finishing replenish yourself with strength by further deep breathing and concentration between eyebrows.

Security Pattern

The following chapter and comments are the outcome of a Sunday morning 'think-in', which started off as a normal discussion on one particular line of enquiry and grew into a fascinating introspective study by the individual members of the group.

Since I started studying relaxation as a means to help solve the difficulties of daily life, I have often wondered why some people are able to adapt to the most exasperating circumstances and are rather the better for it, while others get flustered about the smallest inconvenience. If something complicated crops up they go to pieces, having a nervous breakdown or, worse, they have to be hospitalised. Comparing the imbalanced person with the adjusted members of the rest of the family I found it hard to find the reason. After a time I developed a theory, which I call, for the lack of a better expression, Security Pattern.

People who cope efficiently with their life have some sort of framework or scaffolding made up from an endless variety of things. These are a kind of nucleus of their being, an anchor to hold onto, which gives stability to their life.

A young university professor who is very much in demand for his lectures found travelling all over the world very tedious. The constant change and missing all the little things which make life complete made him feel as if he was losing his personality. He considered giving up the lecture tours, but this would jeopardise his career which was the most important thing in his life. He then found a solution: to take as many of his habits with him to create a home everywhere. Wherever he is, the first half hour is given to breathing and yoga exercises, followed by a cold shower; and before each conference, headstand for ten minutes. No matter how late at night he reads for entertainment, discarding all preoccupations, relaxes, then gives himself positive suggestions for health and ends up by ordering his subconscious to solve the pertinent problems. 'Between these two sessions, every day is completely different, but I feel at home; I am conscious of being myself because my routine never changes.

The building of the emotional Security Pattern starts straight after birth, even to some extent before, when being wanted and expected, all the loving thoughts and preparation, the choosing of a name, the mother preparing with infinite care the layette while dreaming of the wondrous being to come — a girl — beautiful, gracious, loved by everyone, all the unfulfilled desires passing into this future life; or a boy, handsome, strong and clever — the ideals of many men put into one.

Breast feeding is another Security Pattern. It is much more than just nourishing the baby, it is an essential contact, helping to bridge the somewhat brutal ejection from the warm secure womb into the cold world. With every feeding the child feels the warmth and protection. If breast feeding is not possible, and the only reason should be lack of milk, the child should be given its bottle while being held and smiled at and spoken to. Never should the infant be fed lying in bed, or even worse, left alone while drinking.

In heart disease it has been found that, more important than diet and exercises, are contentment and happiness. How much more needed is peace of mind and happiness for the mother-to-be. Tension is the greatest killer of our time and nothing interferes more with the normal functioning of the body. With an unwanted pregnancy there is unhappiness, frustration, anger, desperation. Imagine what all the tension does to the baby in the womb. The poor thing is already handicapped before he is born. If he is lucky the mother instinct will win and he will be accepted, or adoption will give him all the loving care he needs, but he still has the restriction of being rejected within him and this will add more negativeness when he encounters future frustrations.

Unconsciously we look all our life for that happiness we felt as a baby — being touched, held and loved. The unwanted child who receives very little love and affection therefore finds it extremely difficult in later life to know his desires.

There is, like a red thread through all our lives, a deep mysterious yearning; the longing for reunion with God. The pure love of parents is the closest approach to it and satisfies a child completely. A mature person will seek for universal love and get fulfilment through giving rather than receiving as in a harmonious marriage.

Only if this yearning is satisfied do we feel at ease. Quite a number of people have an occasional glimpse of that satisfaction, enough to make this life worthwhile, a few have reached the 'source of longing' and are in a continuous state of contentment.

The child who missed the care of loving parents has missed out on the deep inner satisfaction love provides. He does not know what to look for as an adult and in his search for happiness may try out different things, positive or negative, social or anti-social.

He may seek for satisfaction through great danger; by climbing the Matterhorn or Mt. Everest; by sailing alone around the world; by racing cars; or he may seek a very dangerous job. He may find fame as a star in show business, or direct his urge towards big finance and become obsessed with power and money. Some have to chase after the opposite sex, never satisfied, always changing. Others try out all possible sexual deviations, and some end up involved with drugs and even crime. Whatever man pursues, he will never be truly contented and happy if it does not satisfy his need for love and union with his higher self.

In the average man the Security Pattern is foremost on the personality level and like all personal traits varies enormously, as no two beings are alike.

The Security Pattern being a framework, it is something steady and reliable, always there, part of the make-up of that person. It is there to give meaning to life and project that security everyone so badly needs. This scaffolding is the most effective when it includes all five senses.

Ian was just old enough to join the Marines when the Japanese attacked Pearl Harbour. His unit, which was sent to New Guinea, was almost wiped out, after heavy fighting, by the advancing Japanese. The last few remaining men were taken prisoners, Ian being one of them. The prisoners lived in a world of sheer hell, building the infamous Burma Railway, ill-treated, under-nourished, racked by malaria, dysentery and tropical diseases. Ian survived, but he was in the Rehabilitation Hospital for a long time being treated for malnutrition, tropical ulcers and depression.

After leaving the hospital, with the help of the Rehabilitation Department, he completed his accountancy course, obtained a government job and married. They had two children; generally all was well except for Ian's spells of depression. During these spells of acute depression he had to be hospitalised.

It was after a suicide attempt that the doctor suggested Progressive Yoga Relaxation and exercises. Ian was a regular member of the school and in time he built up his physical and mental health. He is still a member of the Gita and has also taken up his pre-war hobbies of sailing and collecting precious stones. He has joined a yacht club and the lapidary society.

Since enrolling he has not had any nervous problems.

There are all the pleasant things we remember from earliest childhood until we are grown up. Then there are all the good habits we were trained in as children — the more important being the ones we consciously choose ourselves. Security Patterns are only satisfactory if they conform to our sub-conscious ethics. They are part of the success mechanism of our soul.

Ernest is a hardworking bachelor in his thirties. He cannot make up his mind to settle, as he likes to continually change his girl friends. His life seems rather undisciplined and he never attends the same yoga class twice. Some weeks he will come three times, another week not at all, yet he is balanced and harmonious in a somewhat rugged way. His Security Pattern is a daily short Progressive Yoga Relaxation and a visit to the very good old club to which his grandfather and father belonged to before him. A few times a week he dines there with friends, plays chess, or reads. No matter how wild and disorganised his leisure time is, Relaxation and the club give him a helpful Security Pattern.

Different personalities, surroundings and circumstances demand different Security Patterns. In an interview, a prisoner answered my question as to how he had adjusted to prison life: 'Doing my first stretch, I did not want to have anything to do with the others; because of this attitude I had a bad time, was very lonely, miserable, lost and bitter. The second time I conformed with the others, accepted the unwritten prison rules made by the 'boss' (amongst the prisoners). I belonged, took part in all activities and had a standing in the group to which I belonged. Therefore I had no time to be bored or feel alone.'

If a man is in prison for any length of time he must build his props with the hierarchical set-up of the gaol. His self-esteem is built up on props permitted by his fellow prisoners. People in prison, or members of societies, voluntarily conform to ready-made outer props.

The political prisoner on the other hand is not dependent on his loyalty to outer props, his inner word of ideals take their place; as long as he remains true to them they surround him, anchor him, and remain centred.

The three levels of Security Pattern:
Personal:
> The daily routine, work, social order, music accompanying work, Bible, cross, symbols, amulets, match, photographs, jewellery, *ad infinitum.*

Emotional:
> A well adjusted married life, creative work or the right job, being needed, friendships of long standing, pets, gardening, reading, a definite relationship to nature, music and art forms.

Soul level:
> Belief in God, in a higher force, in evolution, in ethics, i.e. that every human being has a place in this world, that he is needed and can fulfil himself. Composing, painting, writing or any creative art form.

All three types of Security Pattern can be acquired at any stage of life. It only needs knowledge about it, determination to build them.

One day a young girl came to see me. We talked about a lot of things and slowly the picture of a very unhappy, rather lost soul emerged. Since dropping out of her art course she had drifted from one cultural society to another, never staying long enough to benefit by the teachings. She came at the oddest moments to see me at home; early in the morning or very late at night. Once she was in such a state of desperation that I kept her with me the whole night putting her to sleep with Progressive Yoga Relaxation. She felt so refreshed in the morning that she joined the school and for a time came to Progressive Yoga Relaxation practically every day. She did not want to go back to university and started work as a helper with a mothercraft association. She became completely involved and is now very contented and happy assisting a nun to look after a group of children.

Going on in life, advancing spiritually, these props can be discarded, one after the other, when not needed any more.

To believe in God,
Man being a God in the making,
Being like Him — alike,
He liking every human being,
All animals, all plants,
Tune into the Universe.

It started with a chance meeting as several of the mothers had not been informed by their children that there was some kind of a function in the school, which would make them late. To pass the time the women had a coffee together in the nearby Expresso Bar. They all enjoyed it so much that there and then they decided to meet once a week. With the time it developed into a daily habit. From the beginning they ruled all domestic talk taboo. Through discussion of everything under the sun they began to identify with the outside world. It could never become boring as the gathering was so conveniently limited in time by the appearance of the children.

The following comments are derived from the 'think-in' mentioned earlier. The authors are two of my co-workers and a member of an advanced esoteric group.

Yoga is my main support at all times, but some of the other props that I find helpful are listed below, not necessarily in order of importance.

Sense of humour and an eye for the ridiculous, especially when I am the butt of the joke or victim of circumstance.

Sense of proportion: I try to keep my priorities listed in proper sequence, and refuse to get fussed over anything that money, labour or time can correct or replace. For other problems I prefer prayer to worry.

Power of suggestion: Before sleeping at night, I relax and suggest to my subconscious mind that I am happy, confident, organised, lucky, or whatever, definitely, I am not, or whatever is needed for the particular problem. Next morning, even if I haven't found the solution, I usually do feel cheerful and confident enough to tackle it afresh, face it squarely, or accept it if it proves insoluble.

Care for my health and safety: For three reasons;
It is easier to get through the chores when feeling energetic.
So that I am not a burden to others through illness or accident.
So that I am well enough to be able to lend a helping hand if it becomes necessary or if asked.

Meeting unexpected behaviour or rudeness in others with curiosity (regarding the psychological angle) instead of an emotional reaction. My curiosity must remain invisible, but trying to trace or imagine possible causes becomes so interesting that the pain or disappointment dissolves. The process can be very instructive. You may discover that something you said, or did, perhaps in all innocence and quite a long time ago, is the cause. Or that it is your personality in general, or some habit or mannerism that irritates or enrages that particular person. If any one of these is the cause, it is salutary for your ego to be taken down a peg, and one can then try to rectify the damage or at least apologise and resolve not to repeat the action. If none of these is the cause and you are in no way to blame you can relax and just feel compassion, or understanding, instead of being hurt.

A creative hobby: Anything that demands concentration, devotion and produces a sense of accomplishment is mental refreshment. It is almost like leaving one's body and entering another world for a few hours that seem timeless.

Escapist occupations for pleasure: Such as reading, meeting friends, sport, theatre, Bridge (or any other card game).

'Mind Stretching' pursuits: Learning or studying new subjects, discussing, debating these.

Friendships: The affection, trust and companionship from these are equally as valuable as props, as are those of husband and children. These are usually far more peaceful and far less demanding.

Emotional independence or detachment: I enjoy (value) many things and friendships, but try not to become obsessed or over-fond of any one activity or person so that I do not depend on it or them for my happiness, satisfaction, or emotional security. I enjoy solitude as much as I enjoy company.

Beauty: Whether in sunsets or a single petal, architectural design, fabric or the lacy pattern of a tree against the sky in winter. A baby, a kitten or any small baby animal. All these kindle the sense of wonder. It is also fun to seek and find beauty that is not immediately obvious to the casual gaze.

The greatest help of all is one that could hardly be termed a prop; it is more like a fortress. It is a growing conviction, acquired through experience and proved, that everything I undertake or everything that happens to me will turn out for the best in the long run, even if it appears to be a mistake or an unwelcome event at the time.

G.P.

A scaffold, a crutch, whether actual or metaphorical, is a prop to give temporary support to a weakness. In man such weakness is fundamentally nothing but his separation from God-consciousness. For this we seek all manner of substitutes, such as the ritual or well-established habits, the familiar, the talisman, the object cherished by one very close to us.

All of these however, can be considered as props because they are really nothing but a refuge, a shelter for our troubled being. We run to them to be comforted, or rather we run to them out of an unavowed, unrecognised fear of that inner void, which becomes magnified when we face the unknown, the new, the out-of-the-ordinary. They are rather moral and mental pain-killers, anaesthetics. Therefore, it is really doubtful if such well-established habits can be considered as 'Strength Pattern', because they are in fact only substitutes, consequently temporary which makes their security value time conditioned.

But then, just as a crutch can help an injured leg or back to regain its strength by offering the chance to exercise it more freely and so bring about a new or renewed degree of flexibility, so can the temporary crutch of a discipline-in-the-learning prepare the way for greater adaptability in everyday life.

The value of discipline does not appear to be so much the thing *per se* as its potential to condition and prepare us in certain ways and to certain degrees. The great merit of self-disciplinary ability lies rather in the fact that with its help we can implement, no matter how simple a resolve, a new habit, under no matter what conditions and circumstances and fortify it by maintaining it as a rhythmic pattern. Such an achievement cannot but strengthen the belief in ourselves and it is only such a belief in one's strength and perseverence which can lead to self-respect.

The person trained in discipline from earliest childhood has a great advantage in adult life over his untrained fellow man. But even the untrained and 'un-spiritual' person cannot help but respond favourably to the elation of 'coming out on top' through one's own will-power and determination, to feel the conqueror, to feel victorious — an enormous boost, like a moral vitamin injection.

Both the moral-pain-killer and the moral-vitamin-booster fit comfortably into a travel-pack which is to accompany us no matter where and into what circumstances. Whereas the first is soothing and pleasurable, but inactive, the second is productive.

I do feel, though, that the success or otherwise of the initial training in discipline as imparted by parents, educators or life itself, will depend greatly, if not entirely, on the basic temperament of the individual. On it would also depend the degree of response, opposition, rebellion, failure.

Reflections on the question of discipline: There is no shadow of a doubt in my mind that the very strict and rigorous discipline which my mother introduced into my life and with which I was brought up has provided me with a metaphorical backbone. From the time I can remember life meant clockwork. A strict routine governed my school years. It occupied every hour of my day till bedtime.

The political situation, which then forced us to leave Berlin, made an abrupt end to this routine, literally from one day to the other and because of this it was almost as though I felt the tiniest of soft spots for Hitler in my heart. I was then very conscious of the despair of my parents and it was this which prevented me from taking advantage of the chaos which arose also as far as my schooling or further education was concerned.

True other disciplines took the place of the old ones almost immediately; having to fit into a new surrounding, establishing new relationships with new people, a new language, new customs, trying to prepare for a career, and all this several times over during the seven years we wandered around Europe until we came to Australia.

But this discipline I did not recognise as a measure of training until many years later; but most certainly it was due to this that I became flexible in adapting myself easily to circumstances and conditions and I did not feel so tied to nationality nor did I feel so uprooted as many others who had to emigrate.

In fact, by the time I arrived here I felt a happy hybrid, unencumbered, a nobody, belonging nowhere and yet, this was the hardest change, as I had to learn to help support the family.

As I write this, it occurs to me that it is much easier to incorporate disciplines into one's life, dictated by an outside agency such as parents, teachers, or life circumstances, than to implement one out of one's own free will, such as a cold shower. When there is no threat, pressure etc., when one is free to turn off the cold tap and turn on the warm, to get up in the morning or turn round for another few minutes and so on, the effort requires much more energy, determination, will-power.

This is why the smaller disciplines are so vital and ever important in the strengthening and balancing process of personalities.

S.G.

Each one of us is protected for the duration of our earthly existence by a 'coat of many colours' — a structure made up of certain experiences in our temporal past which have impressed themselves indelibly onto the various layers of the casing of our soul. Not touching the soul as such, but providing stabilisation, a backbone which helps us to withstand the fluctuations of our life, the many changes in country, housing, influences, people, learning dangers and joys.

Very early in our lives, even before we are born, our parents exert an influence on us by their way of conducting themselves, by their choice of sensual stimulation, be it music or art, or poetry, or simply wind and sea and the beauty of nature. Strong experiences sustained by pregnant women have been found to have an impact on the unborn child. After birth it is the web of ritual (feast days, food, family prayers, winter evenings by the fire and around a piano) which will touch some particular strata of the growing life and there create the first — even if secondhand — patches of the coat of many colours. We get some more from our teachers, but very soon we collect our own. Quite unconsciously at first, we store for later reference those moments and impacts in our life which hold in them for us the strength to counteract stresses, to work like the complementary bow of a bridge and so build our inner fortitude.

What is it that marks a certain experience as suitable in the building of the protective net? It seems to be any experience, encountered with any one of our five senses on both the physical and mental levels which has been completely lived. Living in the present, awareness of the now, awareness of one's personal being, the I am consciousness of the Yogis — these make up the patchwork of the protective mantle. This would explain the discrepancy in the amount of personal 'backbone', personal fortitude which we find in the people around us. The person who is very aware will also be the very strong and yet resilient one. The protective structure is by no means rigid. It will change in its own quality in the course of living and learning more. It will eventually cease to be protective as there will — in the ultimate and ideal situation — be no need for protection and so will become merely buoyant, transcending the restriction of physical life.

We collect the 'patches' on all levels of our five senses. With our sight we drink in a particular combination of lines and colours, a beloved face, the shape of a tree, a sunset, etc. With our ears we mark for future comfort one special voice, the murmur of a creek, the roar of the sea. With our nose we take in and give ourselves to the exquisite perfume of a spice, steam rising from hot earth after summer rain, horses sweating in a sleigh harness, a baby's cleanliness, cedar furniture. Our tastebuds convey comfort with anything from Farex to apricot dumplings, Turkish delight, or the taste of an icicle picked secretly from the roof of a wooden hut. Touch is probably the most subtle of all the senses which take us back into our secret kingdom or makes us draw the protective cloak more tightly around our shoulders. When you watch young children carefully, you find that they will run their fingers gently across an object, completely absorbed, completely part of that object — drinking it in, identifying with it, contemplating rather than concentrating or meditating.

The single units making up our protection can each get out of hand, become over-emphasised and therefore negative. Tradition, ritual, a focus on a habit pattern like personal grooming, a focus on a talisman can become an end in itself, over-ruling the responsibility of living. The stronger the available foci for protection and inner strength, the stronger is the danger of them becoming negative, possibilities for a child to draw 'patches' from his early environment. Tradition can become snobbism, ritual can grow into inflexible conventionalism — all things which turn into 'isms' need to be suspect.

Personal examples:
Throughout a life spent mainly amongst suitcases, in a number of homes, both as a child and as a grown up, marked by an education spent in fourteen schools and a complete changing

of languages, there was one ritual which linked the disorganised and fragmented years like a clasp which holds beads in a chain. Christmas in peace and war was strictly and lovingly observed. It was always celebrated on Christmas Eve in the European manner; always with a tree and candles; always with a Christmas goose or at least a chicken suitably dressed up. Even during the famine in Vienna we managed to trade or beg or 'organise' some kind of bird for the purpose. Always we would dress in evening dress whether it was freezing cold, without heating, or an Australian or Indian scorcher. Always there was the record of Silent Night, Holy Night to be played as the doors were flung wide open to show the lighted tree and the individual tables of presents with gay packages and plates of apples and sweets and home-made biscuits. Always the children had to wait until this moment before they saw the tree or their presents. Even now, my own grown-up children prefer to keep up this mystery. Whatever happened during the year, whatever differences had sprung up between members of the family — during these magical hours on Christmas Eve there was complete union, the certainty that all would proceed according to the ritual of generations. It often cost me a lot of effort, a certain amount of ridicule in foreign surroundings, an unbending attitude towards temptations of holidays with other people etc., but it kept both my own generation and that of my children from losing an identity which helped us grow strong.

In this ritual were incorporated the experiences of every one of my senses. The smell of baking, the spices, the fir tree spreading its exciting smell in a warm room, the candle-wax. The taste of Lebkuchen, a kind of honeycake centuries old. Chestnut puree, the sound of that carol, the sound of the recorders we had to play as children, the sound of the 'Ah!' each child emits when confronted by a glowing tree. The hissing of the sparklers which we still use. The rustle of tissue paper. The sight of the dark fir tree, the glittering ornaments carefully preserved from year to year, some half a century old. The sight of a family absorbed in opening packages, smiling, guileless. The darkness outside the windows, the mellow light from candles, beautiful glasses on the table, women in long dresses.

And touch? The ritual of kissing, a head being close to you to share in a particular surprise — hair brushing your cheek. Your hands finding the texture of a beautiful tablecloth, curving around the stem of a crystal goblet, fingertips touching pine needles — very smooth and yet so strong. As a child, putting one's arms around the cook's ample middle, head against her starched, smooth apron feeling warmth and the smell of cooking.

There are many other 'patches' in each life. A ring we wear that belonged to our ancestors and which from time to time reminds us of a long line of people who coped with life and earned their place in history. A small statue given in friendship, a shell picked up on a beach during a time of complete and immediate happiness. It became important because it remained as a record of a short time of complete living-in-the-present.

B.M.

To Love
To Serve
To Learn and Understand

> Oh Lord, we pray for help
> To love this world
> And every day we live
> To love our brothers
> Yet to stand apart;
> To love you above all
> Within our heart.
>
> Oh Lord, we pray for help
> To serve your cause
> In any way you choose.
> To serve by working
> With the gifts we have
> To serve you without pay
> Because we love.
>
> Oh Lord, we pray for help
> To learn with zeal
> In soul as well as mind,
> The laws of Nature
> And the sacred Truths
> That — learning — we may serve
> And give more love.

To Love
To Serve
To Learn and Understand
Let this be our creed
In years to come.

B.M.

Conscious, Subconscious and Superconscious Mind

That we live a rather unhealthy life is evident. Increase in war; violent, and juvenile crime; theft; drug addiction; suicide; divorce; drop outs from society in general are the pointers.

Man has been driven far away from the natural life he was used to centuries ago and he is becoming more artificial and unnatural in his habits, tastes, food and so on. He has become a slave to unhealthy desires. What is the cause of it?

Poverty? No.
Over-population? No.
The advancement of science? No.
Losing faith in God? To a large extent, yes!
What else? The misuse of the human mind. This is responsible for most of the wrongs which man commits.

To have a healthy mind with which to think rightly, one should have a healthy body. A healthy body does not mean a body with prominent and bulging muscles, but a body free from disease. Therefore, to keep yourself physically fit you must give your body the right kind of food and some exercise. Games, sports or Hatha Yoga can help to replenish energies, mental and physical, which are lost in our sedentary and indoor living.

Since very few spare the time for health it is of little wonder that most of the population are often ill and sometimes confined to bed for days, months, and even years at a time. Only then do they realise what it means to be healthy. Not only is our time and that of those attending us wasted in sickness, but also a lot of money, which could be spent for better reasons.

What is this mysterious and complex human mind? In the course of an incarnation the mind is built up on the foundations of the traits of the higher self, or the individuality, which is the incarnating self, the soul, developing in the course of evolution. The conscious mind is therefore part of the personality, commencing at birth and dissolving at death. Its essence being absorbed by the unit of incarnation, the individuality — superconscious which evolves thereby.

Mind is thoughts, the conglomeration of thoughts past, present, and future. The harmonious co-operation between the conscious mind of the personality and the subconscious mind of the individuality is the greatest power on earth, and is only surpassed by the superconsciousness.

The conscious mind functioning through the physical brain, is essentially the organ for adaption to the environment. The forebrain or cerebrum can be compared to the operator of an electronic brain or any other type of servo-mechanism. It is with the forebrain that our conscious mind thinks 'I' and that we are aware of our sense of identity. With it we discriminate and select, make observations, use our imagination, form judgments, and evaluate sense data.

The conscious mind — personality — is the mind you use every day, with which you speak and think, you reason and discriminate, you make selection without emotion, with which you command. The conscious mind is thought without action.

The forebrain or conscious mind cannot create. For sure the creative imagination issues from there, but the creation product as such, has to come from and through the subconscious. The conscious mind on its own cannot even lift a finger.

It is the job of the forebrain to imagine things, to pose problems, but only the subconscious can solve them; only the subconscious can bring success. The big mistake of modern man is to try and solve problems with the conscious mind, but by its very nature it was never meant to do this. The conscious mind has to think about and study a problem, work at it, be definite about it, but as soon as a decision has been made, the conscious mind has to dismiss all preoccupation with it. The intellect has to leave everything to the subconscious which is the executor and must be allowed to run unhampered by any thought or scheme. The intellect or the conscious mind must surrender completely and be free and unconcerned, taking for granted that everything will come to pass exactly as planned and as decided by the conscious mind in the first place.

Miss E., a telephonist, had one great yearning — to travel, to see the world, to meet different people, taste different foods, breathe different air! Many times she had gone to a Travel Agent and with their help had mapped out a 'dream trip' but she could never quite save enough.

She came to one of the lectures on visualisation; she was sufficiently inspired to work on this technique and she soon found enough determination and impetus to put into action her latest travel plan. Within the same year she went to Japan and came back a transformed person. I still marvel how she did it on her salary. Gone was the shy and self-effacing, over-conservative woman who went her way in colourless anonymity. People began to take notice of her, she could speak with authority on many subjects. When her long service leave was due, she went on a world tour. She has learned to make friends everywhere and keeps in touch with people all over the world, as she has now to stay home to care for her sick and elderly mother.

It is the conscious mind, the objective mind in man, which is different in every human being. Diversity exists only on the level of conscious mind in all living beings of this plane of development. The higher evolved a being is, not just man; the more individualistic he becomes. The conscious mind has developed through evolution, through individualism, and belongs to the earth plane. It is, so to speak, man-made as are languages. That, incidentally, is the reason for the unbelievable multitude of languages, whereas sound issues from the universal mind. This accounts for the universal quality of music — everyone can understand it.

There is no force without the two opposite poles of positive and negative. In a way we can consider the subconscious to be the opposite of the conscious mind. On the conscious level everything is clear-cut, and without interference from the subconscious we would all be cold, precise, infallible — quite repulsively so.

The subconscious gives the impulse to all unwanted and negative reactions. We do not need to be ruled by the subconscious nor do we need to regard it as an enemy. On the contrary, we can use it as our best friend who is eager to help us to advance, but in order to use it as an asset we have to know how it works.

The subconscious is controlled by the conscious mind. It is incapable of independent reasoning by the process of induction. The subconscious, superconscious, soul, and the universal mind are one and belong to the Universe, to God. The subconscious is the mind of the soul. When in stillness it is able to contact our higher mind, we call it conscience. The closer our contact with the subconscious, the happier and more complete we shall be. To be in tune with the subconscious brings out the best in every man; when so attuned inspiration can penetrate from the superconscious region, the region above the conscious mind. If on the contrary the conscious mind and the subconscious are out of harmony with each other we have a split personality.

Being part of the soul's expression, the subconscious mind is the same in all humans. It is the region of the instincts and emotions, and is that wonderful part of you which regulates the beating of your heart, the breathing of your lungs, and all processes of digestion and assimilation. The subconscious is ever active by carrying out and following orders.

It is the subconscious which brings out the magic power of your mind and you must be aware of this all the time, and never forget it. Form the habit of dictating all your desires to your subconscious, because it will act on your command. It keeps a faithful record of all you have said, felt and done in your life. It records things your conscious mind did not even notice. The limits of its power are unknown; it never sleeps and will come to your support in times of great trouble, helping you to do what seems impossible.

When properly used you can achieve whatever you may choose to put your mind to, but beware, and desire only that which is worthy of a spiritually evolving human being. The subconscious cannot discriminate between good and evil and will fulfil your every wish, if the emotional impact is strong enough.

Fakirs and Yogis make use of the power of the subconscious to gain their extraordinary control over their bodily functions. They can sit naked in deep snow and still keep warm. They can walk over glowing coal, can lash their body with a strong whip and stick long needles through any part of it. They do astounding things and have complete mastery over their physical resources.

Give commands to your subconscious and it will never fail to obey, if the order is clear and simple and given with deep feeling. The stronger you feel about something, the more you accelerate its realisation.

The subconscious can only be reached through visualisation. To address the subconscious in words is like speaking to a child in a foreign language; to reach the small child's mind you must use sign-language. It is the same with the subconscious; we actually think in pictures not in words. Our only mistake is to think so quickly that the picture does not have enough time to make a clear and precise impression on the subconscious.

He was tall and fair with a pleasant manner. His name was Dennis and he had come to discuss his problem with me.

For the last few years he had hoped for promotion in his job but somehow he had always missed out.

In his private life Dennis was indecisive and unsure. He'd met a girl whom he would like to marry, but was too afraid to commit himself in case he could not adequately provide for a future family.

I started Dennis on Progressive Yoga Relaxation. Later on, more advanced breathing exercises, visualisation, and suggestion were added. He stuck to the programme for some weeks only, then he stayed away for a while but suddenly appeared again to take up his disciplines where he had left off. This was the start of his adjustment. He had made the first major formative decision and had faced his own shortcomings instead of blaming his surroundings. He worked conscientiously and got results. He married his girl on the strength of his promotion, he started to travel for his firm, he enjoys meeting people as an equal and whenever he comes to the school for a refresher course now, it is a pleasure to see the transformation.

The subconscious dates back to the very beginning of man, to that time in evolution where, as yet, he had no speech, hence no language. Modern mind in its 'mechanical' functioning operates no differently from that of primitive man, who thought in pictures before the advent of language. Returning to his cave and tribe after a hunt, the only way he could convey his experiences was by drawing pictures in charcoal or chisel them on the wall of his cave.

The subconscious will understand every clear picture and act upon it. Knowingly or unknowingly all great and successful men and women in this world have made use of this fact which has been rediscovered by modern psychology as a new idea. This idea is the realisation that what you picture in your mind will eventually come to pass in your life provided you picture it clearly, confidently, and persistently enough. Without this no one could have ever achieved greatness or success.

As Victor Hugo said: 'Nothing in this world is so powerful as an idea whose time has come'. The time has come for the realisation of the unlimited power of visualisation, one of the greatest ideas in the world today, to take possession also of your consciousness.

Look around you, see happy men and women to whom good things are happening. They get up in the morning expecting good things to happen, and good things DO happen to them. There is a mighty force in the world which scientists call electro-magnetism. Everything in the Universe is electro-magnetic in nature; the laws of attraction and repulsion operate electro-magnetically. Therefore, when you assume a positive or negative attitude of mind you get a positive or negative response. There is no such thing as an accident in life — everything happens in direct accordance with the laws of cause and effect.

Ken was a young medical student on a scholarship and working part time. He was determined to prove the possibility of visualisation. He was so sure of his results that he promised me a drive into the hills as soon as his dream-car had materialised.

Not long after, when I enquired about the progress, he proudly showed me the photograph of an old Rolls Royce.

I could not help thinking a motor bike would have been much more useful.

It took some time before I was asked for a drive and I made quite sure to carry enough money with me to aid any salvage operations, should we get stuck.

The drive was a joy. There is something incredibly powerful about a Rolls, even an ancient one. I realised that in visualising and wanting such a car Ken had achieved more than a mode of transport, more than a status symbol, more than a whim. He had got rid of all the longing of his poor, orphaned childhood, where more often than not, even the strictest necessities were missing.

The wisest men of all ages, the great religious teachers and philosophers — Rama, Krishna, Zoroaster, Buddha, Lao-Tse, Confucius, Christ, Mohammed, The Reformers, Guru Nanek, Mary Baker Eddy, Madame Blavatsky — revolutionised the world with their foreseeing visions.

The Mayan priests, shamans, yogis, healers, and miracle men all knew and know this secret; some work it one way, some another. They would picture in their minds and hearts what they wanted — and what they pictured eventually came true.

Moses imagined himself leading his people to the promised land.

Alexander the Great and Napoleon visualised great conquests.

Shakespeare glimpsed the creation of his immortal writings.

Columbus discovered the Americas with his daring thinking.

Michelangelo not only created world-famous sculptures, paintings, and sonnets, he also conceived the dome of St. Peter's in Rome.

Dunant led mankind a step forward with the idea of the Red Cross.

Karl Marx changed the world with his theories.

Edison pictured the electric light, moving pictures, the phonograph, the electric train, and countless other inventions.

Roosevelt visualised leading his country out of its worst depression.

Alexander Fleming helped in conquering infectious diseases through penicillin.

Rev. Flynn brought medical care to Australia's outback with his Flying Doctor Service.

Churchill saw the allied victory.

Mahatma Ghandi foresaw a free India.

Steinmetz anticipated new uses for electric power.

Today's mathematics and physics depend to a large extent on Einstein's theory of relativity.

Gerard Feinberg, Professor of theoretical physics at Columbia University, New York, with his theory of Tachyons will bring our planet into the class of interstellar travel.

All of these great ideas were and are held as pictured by great and inspired men. They were held resolutely in the mind and converted into action. These ideas were brought to pass by faith, vision, energy, courage and steadfastness of each individual. These men and many others like them, were just human beings like yourself. If they knew how to succeed, so can you.

What made these people great? They visualised themselves successful! They dared to picture great achievements, and the power within, given these pictures to work with, finally brought them into being. You have to think big, to be big.

Reflect for just a moment. Take out of this world everything that has been created by thought alone and you will have nothing left but the sea, mountains, primitive jungle and man. This is the simplest and most graphic way to help you comprehend what the mind of man has done. When the real history of the evolution of the mind is written, it will make the greatest, the most thrilling story of all time, because it will cover all time and every phase of human experience. This story will tell how man required thousands and thousands of years to emerge from the depths of ignorance, superstition, fear, prejudice and wrong concepts.

Mr. C. had hypertension and came regularly every day to Relaxation. He was a gentle, kind man and I grew very fond of him and at last he confided in me; his son David, a medical student, had a Christian girl friend. It was just before Easter so I suggested he invite the girl friend to the Passover feast to meet the whole family. While he appreciated the soundness of the suggestion, he could not see his wife agreeing to it. Mrs. C. was not only understanding, she was enthusiastic. I suspected that she would make the most of the tradition. The Christian girl was very ill at ease and she had difficulty in eating the unfamiliar Passover food.

The relationship cooled down on both sides. The girl fell in love with another co-student and David with the daughter of his mother's best friend.

By now Mr. C. trusted my opinion and we had long talks about equality of man and when at last he realised that I was a gentile it did not matter.

He had many helpful experiences through relaxation, one is so beautiful that I have to tell it, exactly as he told it to me.

'I was dressed in the traditional Talmudic way, with Talith, Yamulkah, Payes and carrying the Torah. I was walking up a high mountainside, the land was arid, much as it is near the Dead Sea. It was early morning, but already very hot. As I climbed up the Talith was such a burden that, after a battle with myself, I dropped it. The path got steeper and the heat increased, and I discarded one thing after another. At last I stood naked on the top and an ecstatic feeling of being one with God pervaded my whole being and I felt love for every creature on Earth, in my joy tears just sprang from my eyes.

I have never been the same since. I do not worry, I do not get impatient, and for the first time in my life I give gladly to non-Jewish causes and my distrust of people, other than Hebrew, has left me.'

You, too, can apply this basically simple idea of visualisation. Open your mind to let it in and you will never be the same again. It will destroy all false concepts and replace them with real ones. It will eventually remove fear and worry from your life, release you from chronic nervous tension, chase the butterflies from your stomach, restore your self-confidence, give you a more positive attitude and enable you to face things you have been running away from for years.

In order to be successful you must make a positive picture of what you want to achieve, and hold it in the conscious until it has sunk into the subconscious. Remember the subconscious will understand every clear picture you convey to it and will act upon it. Don't make a picture of something you do not want. For instance, if you do not want to smoke any more, see yourself in company of smokers and you sit easy and relaxed, without smoking with them. You see yourself in all possible situations, in which until now you used to smoke, but without a cigarette. If you want to get rid of the chronic feeling of tiredness, see yourself doing all your work in an easy, steady way. Always find the positive angle of whatever you want to achieve.

The subconscious mind can acquire knowledge of conditions relating to anything. If you have a problem, put it in your subconscious and wait patiently while it assimilates it and works it out for you, in its own way. In due course with a flowing of ideas and plans, a solution to your problems will be revealed to you and the correct course of action indicated. Be sure to always follow the indicated course to the last letter.

It is possible to give yourself valuable auto-suggestion and through the power of the subconscious, alter your entire life. In this way you can turn sadness into joy, order yourself to perform a certain action at a certain time. Knowing the past, the present and the future, your subconscious can also warn you of danger. You should distinguish a hunch or the voice within from wishful thinking. Once you practise relaxation or meditation daily you will soon begin to recognise a hunch. The difference in feeling cannot possibly be put into words. but you will nevertheless recognise it at once and you need have no fear of being carried away by wrong ideas.

When something impresses you as right you know for sure that it is a hunch. It is something you simply cannot explain.

You have heard people say: 'I had a feeling to do this . . .' or 'Somehow I knew I should do it . . .' These are hunches. There are always people who put everything down to mere chance, but these people, and there are plenty of them, never believe in anything. Ignore the unbelievers. Do not talk about your hunches, just follow them. You will not actually hear a voice, but you will be aware that something is going on within you, and that you must follow it.

Many people think they are not responsible for what happens in their life; they blame other people or circumstances. But you, and you alone are responsible. Had you listened to your subconscious every day in a quiet relaxation or meditation, you would have been warned that things were about to happen and advised to do the right thing. In future therefore, follow your hunches, and your life will be more meaningful through the harmony between the conscious and subconscious mind.

The subconscious mind is also open to receive suggestions from others from the outside, but these penetrate to us in different ways, through the written or spoken word. But they will reach the subconscious only if the conscious mind has totally accepted such suggestions. What the conscious mind believes, it pictures and that is how it makes contact with the subconscious. Suggestions reach the subconscious best when the mind is in a happy frame, relaxed and in harmony. Harmony always means in tune with the elements.

The conscious mind is the mediator of the 'trinity' and controls general thinking and the reasoning mechanism. It is responsible for directing the external activities of our body, and for the programming of our subconscious, by the quality of the ideas it habitually harbours.

The subconscious mind is the seat of the animal instincts and animal emotions, and the controller of the unconscious, automatic bodily activities, such as digestion, heart beat and cell growth. When its natural desires and drives are repressed or denied reasonable expression, the result is some degree of psychological imbalance.

The superconscious mind is the seat of inspiration, idealism, morality and conscience. We might roughly relate the subconscious to Freud's 'id', and the conscious to reason. The superconscious is the spirit mind, and our personal contact with Deity or at least the highest moral and spiritual concept of the race.

These three minds should be one, but as the conscious mind is objective and the subconscious as well as the superconscious are subjective, a common denominator is needed. This common denominator is Love, Altruism, and Sacrifice.

Lower self	Higher self
Personality	Individuality
Conscious	Subconscious

These are the tools of the three levels of the mind which can be used for self-analysis. (To be read horizontally.)

Instinctive Mind	Intellect	Spirit Mind
Lower mind	Middle mind	Higher mind
Subconscious	Conscious	Superconscious
Animal	Man	Super-man
Servant	Master	Teacher
Emotion	Reason	Christ-consciousness
Impulse	Logic	Conscience
Past	Present	Future
Compulsive	Rational	Inspirational
Instinct	Five senses	Inner Sight
Compulsion	Discrimination	Perception
Emotion	Body	Spirit
Individuality	Personality	Individuality
	Concrete	Abstract
Subjective	Objective	Subjective
Memory	No memory	Pre-recognition
Emotion	{ Emotionless { Without emotion	{ Pure love { Compassion

Rules for visualisation to achieve your desires.

Unconditioned beliefs, no doubts.

Not to desire what belongs to someone else, nor that which could hurt another person.

To know exactly what you want, keep it absolutely to yourself.

To persevere till the goal is reached, be it physical, material, mental or spiritual.

Use commonsense, choose things befitting your way of life.   Your acquisitions should be an asset and help, not a burden.

Never ever desire money unless you are a miser loving it for its own sake, wanting it to gloat over by the chestful behind closed doors.   Money is a means to an end, it is very useful for exchange and you should like it, treat it with consideration, but do not have flutters when you spend it.   Give it away with a smile, be on good terms with it, and in your mind ask it to come back — with relatives — do not laugh, I mean it; if you have a pleasant relationship with money you will never be without. Money is something wonderful, making life easier, but it should never be used to hurt anyone.   It should help mankind to evolve.   To build up underdeveloped countries, to ban hunger from this earth and to bring free education to every last child.

If it is a car you want, decide the model, colour, all the gadgets.   Get a catalogue, choose your picture for visualisation.   Have a regular session every day till your mental picture is as clear as the photograph.   Hold it as long as you possibly can then dismiss it.   Behave as if you had already paid for it, it is only a matter of delivery now.   Keep to the rules.   If you have difficulty with making a clear picture, start with something smaller and easier to visualise.

The Heron

Beautiful Heron,
Poised on river's edge
Sunk in your own reflection.

Perfect economy of line
Self-contained, rising
On slender legs
Above the mud

The morning sun
Paying tribute, touching
Your greyness, caressing
The two curves
which contain your being

Two curved lines
Reflecting each other
Drawing apart at the base
Almost converging
To make a slender neck.

Drawing apart
Once more — to define
Your head, and
Finally touching
To complete the form

You seem to wait
Divorced from time
And the noise of city traffic
Passing the bridge
Self sufficient — Quite still.

You reflect what I seek
And when you remember
your worldliness
Spreading your wings
Only the sky
Is your limit.

                          B.M.

Creative and Negative Tension

The most outstanding feature of our age is noise, ugly torturing noise. It is there, unending day and night, a strong background, to our lives. All noise jars the nerves causing man to be highly strung. The experience of going into the city for a day's shopping and returning home feeling quite shattered and exhausted is a common one for sensitive people. Many other things are contributory; for instance large crowds, heavy traffic, overheated offices, the sense of everyone hurrying, but principally the irritation and weariness are due to constant noise.

Irritability creates negative emotions and ruffles the calmness of the soul and even after these have died away the movements continue, and some bring disturbance for hours, or even days. Irritability is very common and people who have overcome anger and bad temper still suffer from it.

Of course, irritation is somewhat superficial, it does not penetrate deeply into a well-adjusted person, but nonetheless it is there. It is better to avoid even a superficial irritation, because it affects us so much longer than we realise. In a heavy storm, it is the wind that first stirs the waves, but the waves will continue to swell long after the wind has died down. Any vibration penetrating the subconscious of man goes much deeper and, therefore, has a much more lasting effect.

Some slight unpleasant feeling which passes in a few minutes, may still produce a vague, lingering irritation and the vibrations continue for a considerable period of time. When such a condition is recognised it can be most effectively removed, not by focusing attention upon it, but by developing consideration for others through yoga relaxation. The first step is always difficult, but once you have taken that step, you have started to progress and you will win.

Tension appears to be caused by outside factors, such as noise, the irritating behaviour of other people and a thousand other things, but it really comes from within; it is something we produce as a result of the non-acceptance of our surroundings.

There are two kinds of tension. The first is brought about by the will to create. It is essential for every human being as it gives the necessary impulse for work. Its effect is a kind of exhilarating, tingling vitality.

This world would be hard to bear without the excitement of the heights of creative tension and its counterpart; leisure, ease and play.

If there is a major challenge in your job you need to focus all your power and concentration on one point to produce creative tension to deal with it.

The whole secret of coping with tension is to know when it reaches danger point and to reduce it through letting off steam. People have their own way of achieving this; coffee, drink, stretching, talking it over with friends, a hot bath, a massage, a hair-do, a walk, sports, etcetera, but these give only momentary relief from stress, like a safety valve. Later it will be explained how Progressive Yoga Relaxation gives permanent relief.

The accumulation of creative tension comes when the creative flow is interrupted through circumstances; by other people or by ourselves. We all know the frustration of such moments. It is even worse when we have new ideas and we ignore them through lack of time, or because we cannot be bothered. We suffer more stress through the sins of omission than from anything else.

Executives often have a creative urge which is greater than their ability to use it, so it gets jammed. The enormous pressure can make them lose their commonsense for the time being. It may result in an explosion of temper, a quarrel, reckless driving, or a lot of other emotional outbursts, which people regret bitterly afterwards, as these always leave a negative residue behind.

There are many things which bring on nervous tension. Some are purely personal, but most apply to all people.

For instance: Total migration, change of continent, temperament, language, climate, occupation and food.

Losing the most important person in one's life.

Changing one's job or disliking it.

The constant pressure of debts such as hire purchases and mortgages.

Living in the home of parents when married or having in-laws staying with one.

Earning much more, or much less, than before and, therefore, experiencing a definite change in the standard of living.

Travelling for work or pleasure, especially when it includes retarding or advancing your usual time for many hours.

Then there are a lot of small stresses which do not matter much on their own, but combined with others make themselves felt. Quarrels, being nagged, too many late nights, change of weather, too much alcohol, coffee, tea and food.

> No matter how much stress and strain the future holds for man he can cope with it as he has the capacity to adjust to anything and enjoy life in all its aspects. He needs to consciously face the situation and study it and then use all available means to bring this adjustment about.

Tension through the will to create is invigorating, uplifting, and feels marvellous — the world is yours for the taking. Tension caused by fear and inferiority complexes is nerve-racking and feels horrible. Sometimes the two merge into each other when inspiration is curtailed by fear; when doubts about efficiency invade the subconscious.

The more we overcome fear the stronger our creative power. Fear-tension is compulsory, compared with creative tension which is voluntary. Both get their strength from the subconscious. It is the same force used positively or negatively.

Tension is the contraction of every cell in the body, and because of this we produce too much adrenalin, which is an astringent and contracts the blood vessels, and brings about the acceleration of the metabolism. This is all right in the case of great physical or mental effort, such as jumping, carrying heavy loads, or concentration, but it is harmful when no special strength is needed.

Of all mammals, the human being is the least adequate in defence or attack. For example, compare mankind with the

69

cat family. Its members are very flexible and have an outstanding sense of balance. Their colouring, with their stripes and spots, camouflages them in their native habitat. They are equally at home on the ground or in the trees, and not only does their thick fur protect them when attacked, but they also have murderous claws and teeth and can see in the dark.

Some animals have enormous strength, such as the elephant, buffalo or rhinoceros. Others are extremely swift and can jump many times their height or leap great distances on the ground or from tree to tree. Wherever you look in the animal world, you will find that each one has some special protective feature to ensure survival.

Man is the only one who has none of these extraordinary physical qualities, but he has the most outstanding feature of all living creatures on Earth — mind or thinking power. For this reason, and only for this reason, has he survived better than any other creature. He has survived and inhabits the whole Earth and he is a threat to every other living creature as well as to all plants and minerals.

His marvellous brain and nervous system make it possible for man to adjust to great heat as well as to extreme cold. He is able to exist deep in the bowels of the Earth, or in the rarified air of the highest mountains. Through the help of science he can now live for weeks in the depths of the sea, or travel in outer space. One of the latest achievements is the placing of a laboratory in orbit around the Earth, where scientist-astronauts do research for up to fifty-two days at a time. I believe it is only a matter of a few years and man will be in contact with many other planets.

The brain and nervous system, which are man's greatest assets and which have made survival possible, are also his most vulnerable features. This century, with all the new machinery, new inventions and scientific progress creates a great problem. More and more people are showing that they are not able to cope with the modern way of living. They are unable to adjust to the demands of our technological age. The rapidity of change makes it impossible for great numbers to adjust psychologically. The results in countless stress diseases such as heart conditions, stroke, stomach ulcer, asthma, chronic bronchial disturbances, hardening of the arteries, hepatic conditions, migraines, sinus trouble, dermatitis, arthritis, headaches, insomnia, and naturally all nervous disorders including breakdowns. Some doctors today are even inclined to consider cancerous growths as having their origin in the emotional disharmony created by the internal atmosphere of tension.

Some people constantly disagree with others; they are displeased with the world in general; they nag and argue; they like things done their way, and refuse to see anyone else's point of view. Through this negative attitude they are tense most of the time, until, their body cannot take any more and it becomes diseased.

Progressive Yoga Relaxation does not just mean supple muscles, an untiring body free from fatigue. It means, acceptance of our surroundings and even more importantly, the priceless ability to be resilient, to bend with the storm, and afterwards to be as upright as before.

As tension is hardening and closing up, so Progressive Yoga Relaxation is softening, expanding and opening up. It prevents emotional blows from sinking in and causing damage. We cannot change other people; we can only be so relaxed that contact with other people, and unfamiliar situations will not arouse tension within us.

As the pressure is increasing all the time and there is very little likelihood of it diminishing, we have to look seriously for ways of coping with the modern environment.

We have to find a method of prevention and cure, which is easy and simple and can be done individually and in groups. This is Progressive Yoga Relaxation.

Most human beings have some complex, or as modern youth so very aptly terms it, a 'hang-up'. Some are conscious of these hang-ups, some are not, but we all have them to some extent. The traumatic experiences date back, in most cases, to the first three years of life, when a child is most impressionable. Little things are very important at that age. Many things can bring about emotional insecurity: the refusal of a much-desired toy; being punished unjustly for an act in which a child sees no wrong; the ill-treatment of one parent by the other and so on.

These painful happenings are buried deep in the subconscious, influencing our behaviour, causing a certain habit pattern connected with the reason for the suppression. The influence of it will stay throughout life, increasing with age. This need not be so, Progressive Yoga Relaxation will relieve anyone who practises systematically for three months, or longer when necessary.

The result may come gently, spread over weeks, as in a dramatic releasing of a repressed emotion by reliving the original experience.

From the first hour of Progressive Yoga Relaxation, the individual will experience results; for instance, getting rid of a strong tension anywhere in the body, migraine, backache, or any other acute or latent pain. The relief of pain and depression will last for only a few hours at first. As the student practises every day the time-extent of relief will increase. After the course of three months the subject will, with very few exceptions, be cured. If, after some months, or even years, there is a reoccurrence of stress the person can start a second course and relieve more subconscious pressure.

Tension is the result of stress and strain and causes contraction of the whole body. The human body is enormously buoyant in spite of being the most wonderful precision machine on earth, but unhappiness and harassing inadequacy cause tension. A tense body functions inefficiently.

Waste matter in the body causes fatigue, excess of it — exhaustion. Exhaustion, in turn, makes you lose interest in life. Apart from that, your sense of humour is low, and you are at your worst in all relationships; intolerant, critical, irritable; in fact a burden to yourself and others.

In a relaxed state the blood circulates to every part of the body taking care of supply and elimination. Each cell is reached by capillary vessels. These are finer than hair, blood vessels intervening between arteries and veins. The part just before the vein takes in the waste matter and carries it through the veins to the heart and from the heart to the lungs from whence it is exhaled as carbon dioxide. Now the clean cell is ready to receive oxygen — life force, from the lungs over the heart through the arteries.

Most functions in the human body are done in astronomical numbers, e.g. the human body produces, during every single second of a lifetime, ten millions of red blood corpuscles, and destroys the same amount. To be healthy, man has to have a perfect blood circulation. Tension, through its contracting quality interferes with a smooth-working blood circulation, and is therefore one of the main reasons of stress and strain diseases.

Technique of Progressive Yoga Relaxation

There are short and long relaxations serving different purposes. Start first with short trial periods, ten minutes at the most. Make them longer and longer until reaching an hour. Do the relaxations a few times a week until you are thoroughly familiar with the technique. From the beginning, the use of the same room, as well as the same accessories, is important. This will install a habit pattern from the first session.

Wear something easy like a dressing gown or a kaftan. If you suffer from cold feet, put on loosely fitting woollen socks. Arrange a blanket into a long four-fold strip on the floor, head facing North.

Use a small cushion for the head and place another one under the thighs. In case of an arched back put a very small one under the curvature. Be warm and cosy, well covered without being tucked in. Let the blanket be loose to avoid pressure.

Wriggle yourself into a comfortable position. Push the chin towards the throat to make sure your head is not tilted backwards, and then ease it.

The whole back has to lie flat and straight from the neck to the end of the spine.

The arms are curved slightly outwards so they do not touch the body.

The hands lie easy, palm up or down.

The feet and knees are just a fraction apart and inclined sideways.

Drop your eyelids softly over your eyes, and smile gently with closed lips.

The position should be comfortable enough to be held for an hour without movement. With time, you will not even blink or swallow.

Never make an effort to relax. Relaxation is the opposite to effort. Be utterly passive, like lying on the beach on a hot summer day, contented and withdrawn, on the borderline of sleep, only just awake enough to automatically go over each part of the body without falling asleep.

Set a date and from then on relax every day at the same time till you have reached your aim. Early morning has proved to be the best time for most people. Take precautions not to be interrupted or disturbed by noise. Therefore close the windows, draw the curtains, lock the door, disconnect the telephone and the doorbell. You can only let go if you are safe from interference. To be called out of a deep relaxation can be a shock and unpleasant.

As soon as you are settled, start with the text. Keep your mind on the subject and be conscious of each part mentioned. Think in slow motion, in a drowsy way, and continue up to half an hour. Then give the suggestion of 'Divine peace fills me' thirty to sixty times. You inhale with 'Divine peace' and exhale on 'fills me'. There should be an easy rhythmical flow to lead naturally into deep silence.

The one hour Progressive Yoga Relaxation is exclusively done for this period of silence. It is during silence that dramatic changes occur through different kinds of outlets. There are examples after this chapter.

Experiences during relaxation prove that insignificant events can make a deep impression on the sensitive psyche of a small child.

In relaxation everything happens on the subconscious level. In the beginning you get rid of the tension accumulated during that day. In every session you penetrate deeper into your subconscious and you let all this unfinished, bottled-up action and repression come to the surface. The further you regress, the deeper you invade your subconscious the more relief you will experience.

There may be recollections of forgotten childhood episodes. The experience will have lost nothing of its original intensity. Even if it is nearly unbearable, accompanied by excessive anxiety, do not interrupt it; go through with it and conquer it. Progressive Yoga Relaxation works on the subconscious —

instinctive mind — soul level. The instinctive mind also covers our bodily functions, such as breathing, digestion, blinking of the eyes, swallowing and so on. The instinctive mind is the great storehouse for all skills, impulses, habits and character traits we have acquired through hereditary and present life experiences.

In the practice of Progressive Yoga Relaxation we learn to tap this mine of information, to recall incidents of long ago. We may re-live disturbing and frightening events which have been buried, as compulsive fear and complexes, in our subconscious. Through wilfully contacting the instinctive mind, fear can be faced. We can then, as mature adults, deal with them rationally and by so doing, get rid of their menace to our peace of mind.

Compulsive jerks of arms and legs may happen, or the rolling of the head from side to side. No matter how odd the movements are, never restrict them. Some persons cry or laugh, apparently without reason. Let it happen, it is relief of a heartache from the long-forgotten past. Others swear and use foul language. Never mind, let it come out, perhaps you got punished for swearing and, so, you repressed it all these years.

It came as a shock, when in one of my Progressive Yoga Relaxations, I swore like a trooper in my native Swiss dialect, which I had not used for years. I never have had the conscious desire to use bad language.

It happens that some people have only vague, undefined experiences. Strangely enough, the results are the same; increase in qualitative living and a happier disposition.

Experiences during Progressive Yoga Relaxation vary tremendously from person to person. Each session differs from the next and there is an unpredictable variety. People may experience from the first long relaxation an unparalleled fusion of physical well-being and expanded spiritual consciousness, bringing about top level functioning during waking hours.

The average man of today is only familiar with two states of being — awake and asleep. The wakening state has different levels; dynamic, creative living or an ever-increasing, hopeless battle to go through the day, or just living an uneventful life day after day till the end.

There are also different grades of sleep; dozing, deep sleep and dreaming. In dozing, sound and smell of the surrounding world still reach the subconscious and trigger off memories connected with that specific sense. In deep, dreamless sleep, the physiological restoration takes place, giving a feeling of health and vigour in awakening. During the dreaming state — REM — the psychological adjustment occurs. Subconsciously man assimilates the experience of the previous day and classifies them for further reference.

Progressive Yoga Relaxation is a third, in-between, state, which finishes off what REM could not accomplish. In our fast-living age much change happens in one day alone and the subconscious is frequently not able to cope with all the difficulties during the dreaming state. The undigested difficulties accumulate and become a serious psychological problem, and if not solved will make the life of this individual increasingly harassed.

After many weeks of Progressive Yoga Relaxation some will experience the fourth and truest state of man.

There exists in every human being a centre which is never disturbed by external circumstances. This innermost, natural state is — the vibration of love in the soul of man. Whoever is able to relax so deeply as to contact soul level will experience an all-pervading sweetness, a state of no-desire — complete happiness. It is felt in every cell of the body — yet it is not of the body — it is being in the present, being part of all things, being without separateness, full of love for the whole world and an infinite understanding of it. This one-ness permeates you and every atom of the Universe — this is the Universe.

Even one small glimpse will take the fear of death away from you and you will, at last, achieve fulfilment of yourself by using all potentialities of your unlimited nature.
If we want to function at that highest possible level where

there is quantitative increase of quality, we have to make sure the subconscious does an efficient job.

This is really what it is all about; thorough absorption of all problems by the subconscious leaves the mind free from worry so as to attend fully to the art of dynamic, creative living.

About a week after finishing your Progressive Yoga Relaxation course it is advisable to use a ten-minute session of relaxation to get rid of the stress and irritancy of the day by day high pressure living or start meditaton. By now you have already achieved a habit pattern in relaxation and you can go very deep in a few minutes. Some days in your life are even more demanding than usual and you may have difficulty in settling. In this case do a longer relaxation.

Quite a number of people dislike doing anything alone. They are more successful in group work. If this is the case with you, look for a yoga school, or a centre, where Progressive Yoga Relaxation classes are held. If you are unable to find such a centre, organise your own group, in which each member holds about five successive sessions of relaxation, and the rest of the time participates in the course. It is essential to have personal experiences in Progressive Yoga Relaxation when holding it.

The motivation for giving Progressive Yoga Relaxation should be a sincere desire to help. Your voice will naturally become low and soothing, soft and slow-motion. Inspiration will set in and guide you to say the right word at the right moment.

In the case of strong reaction; jerking, laughing, crying, you must leave the group and do it alone, so as not to disturb others, and also to gain the most benefit, as a group has an inhibiting effect.

At the end of this book there are more full-length exercises in Progressive Yoga Relaxation to help you along.

Short and Long Relaxations to be Done Alone

The beginning and end of every Progressive Yoga Relaxation, whether it be short or long, should be a ritual — more or less the same. The middle part of the Yoga Relaxation must vary to avoid monotony and yet be familiar enough to be acceptable to the subject's subconscious mind. This middle part ends in silence — no thinking, just lying passively — from one to twenty minutes.

First short relaxation: (ten minutes)

Beginning ritual:

I relax the tongue . . and place it gently behind the lower front teeth . . I part my teeth just a fraction . . and let the lips touch ever so lightly . .

Then I withdraw my senses: I withdraw the sense of smell into the middle of my brain . . I withdraw my eyesight . . my eyes are closed . . and deep, deep in their sockets . . I do not impose on my eyes, I just let them go . . as long as they are completely at ease . . Then I withdraw the sense of touch from everywhere over my whole body . . turning it inwards to rather feel the inside of my body and not the surface . . Then I withdraw my hearing, feeling all noises fade away . .

I inhale deeply and I fill my lungs . . as I exhale I sink deeper, and deeper into myself . . I inhale . . and I sink deeper, and deeper into myself . . I inhale and withdraw more . . and more . . now I am very deep in myself . . in a contented frame of mind.

Middle part:

(interchangeable). My breath has become effortless, easy and rather shallow . . I feel my right arm very limp and easy . . Then I feel the left arm relaxed and at ease . . I feel the right leg very relaxed . . sinking into the blanket . . I feel the left leg sinking just a little more deeply down into the blanket . . Now my chest becomes relaxed and easy . . sort of flat . . and it feels so lovely I cannot help smiling . . I am so quiet in myself and I feel so cosy . . so completely passive . . I am without a thought . . and I drift into silence . . (two minutes)

End ritual:

Now I bring consciousness back to my hands . . I move my fingers . . I am conscious of my feet . . I wriggle my toes . . I blink my eyes very strongly . . I point my toes downwards . . I stretch my arms up in the air and stretch them gently to the utmost . . Now I put my arms over my head and stretch and arch . . then I turn over on my left side and stretch and arch . . Then I roll over to the right side, I sit up and stand up and stretch once more feeling on top of the world and in love with life.

After a few sessions, when you know it by heart you move to the next, slightly more progressive relaxation.

Second short relaxation: (fifteen minutes)

Beginning ritual:

Middle part: I feel my right shoulder easy and relaxed . . I slowly move down the arm . . and as I move with my mind I feel all tension dropping out . . The elbow feels easy and flexible . . the forearm very relaxed . . and I am conscious of my hands being very relaxed and flexible . . I let my mind move a few times up and down the arm . . each time it is a bit more relaxed . . (Repeat the same with the left shoulder, arm and hand).

Consciously my mind moves to the right hip . . my hip is very relaxed and easy . . my thigh is very easy . . the knee is relaxed and easy . . and the calf is utterly at ease . . my foot inclines to the right it is so relaxed . . I let my mind move up and down the leg . . and each time it feels lovelier and more relaxed. (Repeat the same with the left leg).

Then I feel my chest getting easy and flat . . and I am conscious of the solar-plexus in the middle of the body where I sometimes feel butterflies and knots . . I imagine opening a tight belt . . and I enjoy the ensuing comfort and ease . . I am so relaxed . . I just have to smile . . I take the smile into the solar-plexus . . and from there to the whole body . . and smilingly I glide into silence. (Each day add a minute till you reach five minutes).

End ritual:
When you are fluent in this second relaxation progress to the next one.

Third short relaxation: (twenty minutes)

Beginning ritual:
Middle part: My right shoulder becomes very heavy . . my upper arm is at ease and very heavy . . my forearm is relaxed and very heavy . . my hand is relaxed and very heavy . . my whole arm feels very heavy . . heavy as lead . . (Repeat with the left arm).
My right hip feels very heavy . . and my right thigh very relaxed . . and very heavy . . my calf is easy and very heavy . . my foot feels very relaxed and very heavy . . my whole right leg feels heavy as lead . . very, very heavy . . (Repeat with the left leg). My legs feel as heavy as if they were under a concrete slab . . My chest feels very heavy . . my abdomen feels very heavy . . my whole body feels very, very heavy . .
I feel the heaviness lift slowly from my chest . . then the heaviness disappears from the abdomen . . then my right arm feels light . . my left arm feels light . . my right leg feels very light . . and my left leg is very light . . Now my whole body feels light . . and it is getting lighter . . and lighter . . floatingly light . . weightless . . and I float into silence . . (Each day extend it till you reach eight minutes).
End ritual:

Fourth short relaxation (Twenty-five to thirty minutes)

Beginning ritual:
Middle part: I relax my throat . . and I feel it expand . . and there is only ease and lightness in the throat . . and

80

I feel that ease and lightness in my lips . . and I feel
the lightness spreading over my right cheek . . then my left
cheek feels light and easy . . then my whole face feels
relaxed . . and the skin feels smooth and lovely . . I
feel that ease in the forehead . . Now I feel the scalp
relaxed and easy . . then I feel a lightness in my neck . .
and I feel a wonderful ease and lightness in my back . . and
I consciously sweep down the right side of the back . . then
I sweep down the left side of my back . . Then I relax the
chest . . and I relax the solar plexus . . I relax the right
shoulder . . and from the shoulder I sweep down the whole
right arm to the hand . . my right hand feels very light
and easy . . I relax the left shoulder . . and from the
shoulder I sweep down the whole left arm to the hand . . my
left hand feels very light and easy . . I relax the right
hip . . and from the hip I sweep down the whole leg to the
foot . . my right foot feels light and easy . . then I relax
the left hip . . and I sweep down the whole left leg to the
foot . . My left foot is very light and relaxed . . Now
my whole body is very relaxed . . and easy . . Every
bone in my body is relaxed . . and all my joints are light
and easy . . every muscle feels relaxed . . and I imagine
my nerves like silken threads all over the body so relaxed . .
I cannot help smiling and smilingly I drift into silence (ten
minutes).

End ritual:

After you have done this relaxation for a while, you can
start with the long relaxation, but in the beginning do only
ten minutes of silence increasing as it comes naturally to you.

First long relaxation (forty to forty-five minutes)

Beginning ritual:

As in Short Relaxation.

> Direction: This time do the whole relaxation with a total
> awareness of breathing all the time. Breathe deeply
> without the slightest strain and then as you exhale, very
> consciously send prana — life-force — in a straight line
> to the part concerned, the part you are conscious of.
> When you breathe do not force, just take a gentle breath
> and without effort and very gently breathe in to the

count of four and exhale to the count of four (approximately).

Middle part: I go directly from the lungs in a straight line to the spine . . inhale . . exhale, I go through the whole length of the spine . . inhale . . exhale, I go through the whole length of the spine . . my whole spine is wonderfully relaxed . . and my whole back is completely relaxed

Inhale . . exhale, and I go in a straight line to my throat . . inhale . . exhale, I go to the lips . . inhale . . exhale, and I go to the nose . . inhale . . exhale, and I go to the right cheek . . inhale . . exhale, and I go to the left cheek . . inhale . . exhale, and I go to the right eye . . inhale . . exhale, and I go to the left eye . . inhale . . exhale, and I go to the right ear . . inhale . . exhale, and I go to the left ear . . inhale . . exhale, I go to the whole of the brain . . inhale . . exhale, I go to the back of the head . . inhale . . exhale, I go to the back of the neck . .

Inhale . . exhale, I go to the whole chest . . inhale . . exhale, I go to the solar plexus . . inhale . . exhale, I go to the abdomen . . now my whole head and my whole trunk is wonderfully at ease and relaxed . . very relaxed

I go in a straight line to my right shoulder . . inhale . . exhale, right upper arm . . inhale . . exhale, right elbow . . inhale . . exhale, right forearm . . inhale . . exhale, right wrist . . inhale . . exhale, right thumb . . inhale . . exhale, right middle finger . . inhale . . exhale, right little finger . . now my whole right arm is very relaxed.

I am very peaceful . . at ease . . and I have a delightful feeling of confidence also . . and ease . . and of security . . somehow I feel so very easy that it makes me very strong . . strong and fearless . . and I feel good . . Now I go to the left shoulder . . inhale . . exhale, left shoulder . . inhale . . exhale, left upper arm . . inhale . . exhale, left elbow . . inhale . . exhale, left forearm . . inhale . . exhale, left wrist . . inhale . . exhale, left thumb . . inhale . . exhale, left forefinger . . inhale . . exhale, left middle finger . . inhale . . exhale, left ring finger . . inhale . . exhale, left little finger . . inhale . . exhale, left little finger . . again I feel the whole left arm wonderfully relaxed and easy . . I feel the blood circulate in my left arm . . and my ease is increasing . . and I feel lighter . . and easier . . and more contented . .

Now I go to my right leg . . inhale . . exhale, right hip . . inhale . . exhale, right thigh . . inhale . . exhale, right knee . . inhale . . exhale, right calf . . inhale . . exhale, right shin . . inhale . . exhale, right ankle . . inhale . . exhale, right heel . . inhale . . exhale, right instep . . inhale . . exhale, right big toe . . inhale . . exhale, second toe . . inhale . . exhale, third toe . . inhale . . exhale, fourth toe . . inhale . . exhale, little toe . . now my whole right leg is very relaxed and very much at ease . . and I can feel the blood circulate down and up . . downwards, it feels stronger than upwards . .

I can feel that rhythmical coming and going of the blood . . and I feel easier and somehow flatter and I feel more and more as though I am expanding . . and I am very contented with myself . . very much at ease . . with myself . . feeling a bit like a cat purring . .

Then I go to the left leg . . inhale . . exhale, left thigh . . inhale . . exhale, left knee . . inhale . . exhale, left calf . . inhale . . exhale, left shin . . inhale . . exhale, left ankle . . inhale . . exhale, left heel . . inhale . . exhale, left footsole . . inhale . . exhale, left instep . . inhale . . exhale, left big toe . . inhale . . exhale, second toe . . inhale . . exhale, third toe . . inhale . . exhale, fourth toe . . inhale . . exhale, little toe . . now my whole left leg is completely at ease and wonderfully relaxed . . and again I feel that rhythmical coming and going of the blood . .

I can feel ease everywhere in my body . . in all my bones . . I can feel ease in every joint . . in every ligament of the joints . . in every cartilage of the joints . . I feel that wonderful ease in every muscle . . and in every tendon . . I feel it in every single nerve of my body . . and I feel it in every blood vessel . . I feel it in the lymphatic system . . and I feel it in all my skin . . in fact there is not a cell in my body which does not feel very relaxed and easy . .

I am especially aware of my hands . . and I can now understand the healing power of hands . . everyone can do healing with their hands . . hands are the most wonderful instruments . . there is nothing like them on this earth . . actually there is nothing that machines do which cannot be done by the hands . . hands are not just to do things . . to have dexterity . . to be very clever . . hands should be used to do good . . to caress . . to support . . to guide . . to console . . to fortify . . to be helpful . . to reassure . . and especially to heal . . and when they are sometimes used to punish, it should always be done with kindness . . and even if the grip has to be firm, it should still have some tenderness in it . . Now I give myself to stillness . .

Silence for ten minutes . .

End ritual:

Second long relaxation: (fifty minutes)

Beginning ritual:
Middle part: After the ritual let your breath become fully automatic. Direct your consciousness to that part of the body which you are relaxing and feel a tingling sensation. In some parts it is easier to feel than in others. You may consider it helpful to breathe twice for the same part. As this relaxation will take longer, leave the part relating to the hand out (as described in the final paragraph of the previous relaxation).

Slowly increase the period of silence.

End ritual:
After having mastered the second long Relaxation, progress to the third, even more advanced form.

Third long relaxation: (fifty-five minutes)

Beginning ritual:
Middle part: As soon as your breathing is automatic direct your consciousness to each part of the body as in the second long relaxation. But this time you feel the blood pulsate in

each part. Before the silence you very slowly repeat: —
'Divine Peace fills me' about twenty times.

Silence up to twenty minutes.

End ritual:

If you want more variety alter the group scripts into personal
Progressive Yoga Relaxation.

Short and Long Group Relaxations

Group-relaxations can vary much more in all three parts than the Progressive Yoga Relaxation to be done alone.

First short group-relaxation (ten minutes)

Beginning ritual: Take an easy position, feet slightly apart, arms comfortable, feel your back melting into the ground and all the tension leaving you.

Middle part: Your body is very heavy, at ease and warm . . listen to your heart . . it is beating steadily . . and regularly . . As you listen to your heart . . you feel its beat in the whole body . . It feels as though you are on a boat . . on a quite calm sea . . with the water lapping against the sides . .

The inhaling and exhaling is like the waves . . they are gently rocking you . . The rocking continues in your mind . . and as you rock . . one after the other the negative emotions are dropping out of you . . frustration . . sorrow . . depression . . heartache . . worries . . resentment . . and all the rest . .

You feel serene and contented . . You feel so wonderful you would like the whole world to enjoy it with you . . and out of the depths of your heart rises a great lightness . . and you feel it flow in a continuous steady stream through your whole body . . and all the time you feel lighter . . and lighter . .

Silence (two minutes)

End ritual: It is time to stop your relaxation, move your fingers, wriggle your toes, come back to this world feeling refreshed and invigorated.

Second short relaxation (ten to twelve minutes)

Beginning ritual: give yourself completely to relaxing. It is quite right to wriggle around a bit to find the most suitable condition, so that from the very beginning you feel at ease.

Middle part: There is a languidness around you which makes it easier to let go . . and with very big and broad movements of your mind you sweep down along the spine . .   from the back of the head down . . you sweep out whatever tension might still linger there . . Feel it move out through the legs . . from the hip right down through the leg . . and out through the toes . .

Once more from a little higher . . from the back of the head . . again you sweep with a mental gesture . . into the right shoulder . . down the right arm . . and out through the fingers . .

And again from the head . . to the left shoulder . . down the left arm . . and out through the fingers . .

And again a big sweeping movement . . very light from the crown over your face . . the throat . . the chest . . the diaphragm . . the abdomen . . and once more down through the legs . . and out through the toes . .

The whole body feels relaxed and clean . . It is a free feeling . . a light feeling . . a soaring feeling . . You give yourself to this great enjoyment of feeling so light . . free . . relaxed.

Silence (three minutes)

End ritual:

Third short group-relaxation (twelve to fifteen minutes)

Beginning ritual: throat relax . . tongue relax . . place the tip of the tongue behind the lower front teeth . . part your teeth a fraction . . your lips are softly closed. Withdraw the sense of smell into the middle of the brain . . let the eyelids drop gently over the eyes . . turn your eyesight inwards . . turn the sense of touch inwards . .

withdraw your hearing . . leaving only a fraction, just enough to hear the suggestions . .

Middle part: Listen to the silence around you . .
Listen to the silence within you . .
Listen to the softness of your breath . .
Listen to your heartbeat . . steady and calm . .
Listen to the calmness in your whole body . .
Feel the calmness in your legs . . in your arms . .
There is an ease in your whole back . .
The chest is soft and relaxed . .
The abdomen is flat . . and relaxed . .
There is peace in your face . . great peace . .
There is deep peace in your whole body . .

Silence (five minutes)

End ritual: Bring your consciousness in your hands, open and close your fingers. Wriggle your toes, point your toes to the ground. Blink your eyes very quickly and stretch your arms up and stretch the whole body, start gently and continue to the utmost. Turn on the left hip and arch, turn to the right hip and arch, sit up, stand up and feel on top of the world.

Fourth short group-relaxation (seventeen minutes)

Beginning ritual: as in third Progressive Yoga Relaxation.

Middle part: Your body is very relaxed and easy. The right arm is getting very heavy . . heavier . . and heavier . . now the left also is getting heavier . . and heavier . . Then both legs are getting heavy . . heavier . . and heavier . . The whole body is very heavy . .

After a while the heaviness is leaving and you feel light and warm . . You have a feeling of expansion . . and greater lightness . . then you feel your breath expanding . . your whole body is breathing . . and you feel the air sweeping from your feet to your head . . then the current changes . . and you feel the air from the head to the feet . . the head, feet and hands feel very light . . The air is very invigorating . . every pore in your body is tingling . . you feel wonderfully vitalised . .

Now you feel the expansion of the mind . . it feels very real . . and the mind is expanding further . . and further

. . you are not an entity any more . . you are part of this world . .

Silence (seven minutes)

End ritual: as in the third.

First long group-relaxation

When you do relaxation it is very good to condition yourself to it, to realise that you do this with your own free will, and that you want to make the best of it, you want to achieve the best results so just for the moment give some suggestions to yourself, say: 'I go as deep as I can and I will go deeper today than I have ever been before,' or something of that kind, formulate it in your own way, but do it positively, it is always good to give orders to your subconscious.

Then you check each part of your body, making sure that each part is at ease, because from now on you should not move a hand, a foot, or even an eyelid, you should be completely still. As long as you move, you cannot really relax.

So I will take you inside, away from your senses, and you withdraw your sense of smell, you withdraw it in the middle of the brain, your eyes are closed, deep . . deep in their sockets . . and you withdraw your eyesight . . and you turn it inwards . . you withdraw your sense of touch . . turning it inwards . . taking it away from the surface of the skin . . Then you withdraw your hearing . . leaving only a tiny bit, just enough to hear the suggestions.

Now you inhale and with every breath you go deeper . . deeper . . and deeper into yourself . . inhale and with-draw deeper . . and deeper . . inhale . . and withdraw deeper . . and deeper . . you are in a world of your own, you feel rather alone, I am only a voice, you are not concerned about anything else only yourself . . you feel your tongue . . you let the tongue go limp and soft, and easy . . then you place the tip of the tongue behind your lower front teeth, part your teeth, just a bit . . and feel the jaw very relaxed . .

Then you observe your breathing, it has already become fully automatic . . and you are the observer, the onlooker . . you do not regulate your breath . . you do not do anything about it . . you only observe it . .

Try to consciously take in the relaxation you do now . .
try to be aware of it . . how your eyes are very relaxed
. . feel that coolness in the head . . and feel that lightness in the neck . . there is no pressure . . there is only
ease . . ease really everywhere . . your chest is wonderfully easy, and rather expanding sideways . . and the breath
is just streaming in . .

There is no heaving . . there is no straining . . no
forcing . . your diaphragm is moving automatically . .
remember wherever there is a vacuum, air goes . . and so
you make a vacuum and the air streams in . . the diaphragm
sinks down, closes the vacuum and the air goes out . . feel
that automatic action and feel how easy it is . . and that
is actually how we should breathe all the time . .

Then you feel your throat . . and you feel that expansion
in the throat . . there is only ease and lightness in your
throat . . and you feel that ease and lightness in your
lips . . and you are conscious of the beautiful shape of
your mouth . . of that arched upper lip . . and of the
full soft lower lip . . and it is so pleasant . . that just
the beginning of a smile starts on your lips . .

And you feel that smile spreading over your whole face . .
you feel that smile going over your whole right cheek, and
you feel that smile in the right eye . . and you feel that
smile in the right temple . . and you feel that smile of the
left cheek . . in the left temple . . and in the left eye
. . and you feel that ease and the smile in your forehead . . now you feel your whole face beautifully relaxed
. .

When you are tense you push all your muscles in the face
towards the nose . . when you relax you undo this and the
muscles go back where they should be . . they go into
place . . and it is a wonderful feeling . . you also look
much younger . . and very serene when you do this . .
you can actually feel it, you feel all the wrinkles smoothing
out and you feel that wonderful ease in your face . .

Then you feel that ease in your forebrain . . and you
feel that ease in the middle brain . . and you feel that ease
in the little brain in the cerebellum . . Now you can feel
the blood pulsate in your brain . . and you feel the pulsation

of the blood, deep in your right ear . . deep in your left ear . . you feel the scalp very relaxed and easy . . you feel again that stretching of the skin, from the middle of the scalp outwards . .

And you feel that ease in the back of the neck . . the back of the neck, the back of the head are very sensitive to tension, so we will especially work on this . . and you imagine you go out to the right shoulder . . and you slowly move with your mind inwards, to the base of the neck . . and up the neck on the right side . . and up on the back of the head till you come to the crown . . and then you move very gently down again . . down the head . . down the neck and over the shoulder . .

As you go again, you can feel the tension dropping out, as you go it just leaves and there is a wonderful easy feeling up to the crown, and again down and over to the shoulder . . and we do it a third time . . Slowly move in and up the neck . . up the head . . and slowly down and over to the shoulder . . now it is already much easier . .

We do it on the other side . . from the outside of the left shoulder, you go in and up the left side of the neck . . up the left side of the head till you come to the crown . . and you go down again . . down the neck . . and down over to the shoulder . . and as you go you feel all the tension leaving . . and a wonderful feeling of freedom as you move up and up to the crown . . then slowly down and over to the shoulder . . and once more slowly up and it is wonderfully easy, the shoulders are very relaxed . . and up and up to the crown . . and slowly down and out to the shoulder

Now you feel the back of the head very relaxed and easy . . To make sure all tension has gone, you imagine tiny little men with buckets and brushes going in and scrubbing every nerve . . and rinsing with fresh water every part of the back of the head . . they scrub and rinse . . can you imagine all these little green men working very hard on every muscle, on every nerve and scrubbing all the tension away . . and there is only cleanliness and ease everywhere in the back of your head . . in the back of your neck . .

Now your head is so relaxed . . your neck is so relaxed . . sinking deep into the cushion . . wonderfully relaxed and easy . . and your smile goes automatically in the back to the head . . it feels so good . . and you know you will feel easy the whole week . . you will be able to cope with every situation in your life . . and you will enjoy every day . . you will enjoy whatever you do . . from morning till night . . you will wake up happy and go about the day in contentment and ease . . enjoying your resting . . These three should always be equal, one third of your time should be leisure, entertainment, pleasure . . one third should be work . . and one third should be rest . .

Now a lovely cloud is coming and carrying you away up in the sky, high up where the sun is always shining . . and you float on your cloud . . looking down, seeing all the hustle and bustle of the city, feeling a great compassion with mankind realising that most of our worries are self-made . . You realise how often you worry about things which never ever happen . .

And you feel prana streaming into you . . everything is light and easy . . and all your sorrows . . all your worries are dropping out of you . . you are so relaxed . . so easy that nothing can stay . . everything just has to drop out . . and you get very empty . . you empty out all the negative emotions, sadness, and heartache, and you will be very careful . . to replace them with positive emotions, and remember that you are unlimited if you make it so . . you limit yourself, no-one else does it to you, and you can get rid of the restriction and be unlimited . . and you feel this up there in the sky . . you feel that there is no end to your possibilities . . everything is possible . . and with that lovely feeling, you stay up there . . do not think . . just float about and you are at ease . .

Silence from ten to twenty minutes . .

Now very consciously you float down on your cloud . . now you are down, and you are conscious of your body again. You wriggle your toes, you are conscious of your hands, conscious of every part of you, open your eyes, go up with your arms, and reach and stretch, turn over to the left side, stretch and arch, and be very conscious of your lovely, flexible body, and over to the right side and be conscious of your wonderful mind. Do not lie on your back, come up from the

92

right side, help with your hands, but come up from the right, and stand up and stretch in all directions . . get all the drowsiness out of you so that you are wide awake, on top of the world.

Second long group-relaxation

Try and remember that the less you try to relax, the less you work at it, the easier it is. The more passive you can make yourself, the more you can follow my voice, my instructions, the more likely you are to get to that borderline between sleeping and waking, which is very deep relaxation.

If you find yourself drifting over into sleep, don't fight it, it doesn't matter, you might not remember a few sentences that have been said, but your subconscious will take it in just as well, and the benefits will be the same.

Relax your jaw . . relax your tongue . . think of your tongue as a very large, very strong muscle, when it is relaxed it expands, it fills the cavity of your mouth, and you feel the tip of your tongue resting just inside your front teeth, just touching . . Relax your teeth . . relax your gums . . relax the roof of your mouth . . relax your throat, so that there is no tension, no restriction in your throat . . Relax your mouth . . your lips . . feel your lips becoming fuller, softer, the shape of your mouth changes as you relax . .

Try and smile, just a little bit . . It is a nice day . . it is peaceful in here and warm under your blanket . . you are comfortable . . For an hour or so you have nothing to do . . nothing to think . . nothing to organise . . you simply give in . . it is nice to look forward to and it is easy . . then you smile . . just a bit . . The moment you smile to yourself . . not a polite conventional smile . . not a smile that anyone sees . . simply one of contentment . . the corners of your mouth turn up instead of down . . and that smile changes your face . . takes away the lines of tension . .

Your cheeks relax . . right back towards your ears, and then up towards your cheekbones . . Be conscious of the bony structure of your face . . feel your cheekbones supporting the flesh and muscle that make up your cheeks . .

Relax the skin around your eyes . . all the tiny little lines . . relax your eyeballs and feel them sinking down very deep into their sockets . . Relax your eyes . . and feel them sinking down very deep into their sockets . . Relax your eyelids . . they are not pressed down, they do not flutter . . they are closed gently and lightly, like the wings of butterflies, and the darkness behind your closed eyelids is peaceful . . velvety . . friendly . . and you can feel the smile that started on your lips even underneath your closed eyes . .

Relax your eyebrows . . feel them like two arches . . one above each eye . . quite separate with a space in between and the space is flat and relaxed without a frown . . Relax your forehead . . feel the lines disappearing . . feel your forehead expanding in all directions . . becoming broader and wider . .

Relax your scalp . . be conscious of the blood circulating underneath your hair . . moving and tingling . . making your scalp flexible . . relax the back of your neck . . that part high up on your spine . . on the junction between your spine and your skull . . the part which collects all the tension . . all the frustration . . all the resentment during the day, all these things seem to come together like a tight knot at the back of your neck . . until eventually, you get what is called a pain in the neck . . It is a very real thing, it is tension built up and collected . . Try and dissolve the accumulated ball of tension . . Relax the back of your neck . . feel your neck becoming longer and straighter . .

Relax the muscles between your neck and shoulders . . and feel your shoulders expanding, spreading out . . sinking down . . Relax your shoulderblades . . relax your spine . . start with the very top of your spine and take your mind very slowly down through all the vertebrae . . through the small of your back . . and the base of your spine . . feel your spine becoming longer and flatter . . losing all tension . . all pain . .

Then take your mind within . . up to the top . . this time to your right shoulder . . and use it like a flat hand to gently stroke down the right hand side of your back . . the way you would stroke the fur of an animal . . and as you move slowly down the right hand side of your back you feel

94

all the muscles . . fibres . . and nerve-ends flattening out . . smoothing out . . losing that tension . . relaxing . .

Take your mind to the left shoulder . . and once again use it in a broad sweep and sweep down the left hand side of your back, flattening . . smoothing out muscles . . nerves . . fibres . . right down . . feel your back supported by the blanket underneath you . . leaning against the ground . . finding support . . enjoying that feeling of support . . giving in to it more and more . .

Relax your buttocks . . relax your hips . . feel your hip bones expanding . . relax your tummy muscles . . feel your tummy caving in, as the muscles relax . . Relax your inner organs . . they are suspended now without pressure . . without restriction . . working efficiently . . easily . . without discomfort or pain . .

Relax your waist . . relax the muscles across your chest, feel your rib cage expanding sideways, becoming broader and wider . . feel how your heart and lungs can work efficiently . . easily without any tension or restrictions . .

Relax your right arm . . upper arm . . elbow . . forearm . . wrist . . palm of your hand . . back of your hand . . and all the fingers on your right hand . . one by one . . thumb . . forefinger . . middle finger . . ring finger . . little finger . . Your whole right arm and right hand are very still . . heavy and relaxed . .

Relax your left arm . . upper arm . . elbow . . forearm . . wrist . . palm of your hand . . back of your hand . . and all the fingers on your left hand . . one by one . . thumb . . forefinger . . middle finger . . ring finger . . and little finger . . your left arm too is relaxed and heavy and very comfortable . . both hands quite still, without action . . without movement . . it happens very rarely, even in sleep we usually clutch with our fingers . . we move our hands to make fists . . very rarely are our hands and fingers completely still . . their movement arrested, all their potential skill and possibilities resting . . Be very conscious of your still hands for a few moments.

Relax your right leg . . thigh . . knee . . calf . . ankle . . footsole . . instep . . and all the toes on your

right foot one by one . . big toe . . second . . third
. . fourth . . and little toe . .
Relax your left leg . . thigh . . knee . . calf . .
ankle . . footsole . . instep . . and the toes on your
left foot, one by one . . big toe . . second . . third
. . fourth . . and little toe . .

Both feet . . both legs . . relaxed and very heavy . .
Feel how they get heavier and heavier . . sinking down
towards the ground . . supported by the ground . . resting quietly . . easily . . the trunk of your body very
still . . very heavy . . your hands . . your arms . .
relaxed and heavy . . the contact between the ground and
your arm becoming stronger the more you relax . . your
neck is quite relaxed, your head heavy and relaxed, and your
face still with that little smile . . serene . . peaceful
. . soft . . smooth . . and young, like the face of a
child that is asleep . .

Concentrate for a moment on your breathing . . how
easily your breath is going in and out of your chest . . there
is no struggle . . no fighting for breath . . it flows in
and out of your lungs . . easily and gently. There is a
definite rhythm in your breathing, it is a rhythm peculiar to
yourself, it is like a signature tune, it belongs to you, and you
can use it to relax yourself even more . .

Concentrate on the rhythm of your breathing . . take your
mind deep inside you . . Be aware of the gentle rising and
falling of your chest . . expansion and contraction . . a
rhythmic movement . . feel your whole being gently rock
by the movement of your breathing . . by the rhythm of this
expansion and contraction . . it is like the tides . . it is
like everything else around you . . everything in the Universe runs in cycles, according to a certain rhythm . . day
and night . . sun and moon . . the tides . . months and
years, all moving rhythmically, changing, ebbing and flowing,
expanding and contracting, and we do the same . .

When we become aware of this rhythm we can use it, to
find strength and stability and harmony, right within ourselves
. . without outside agency . . concentrate on the rhythm
of your own breathing . . feel yourself gently rock by the
movement of your chest, like a child in a cradle, finding in this
movement, comfort and peace . .

Concentrate more and more on that rhythm then realise that your own rhythm, your own harmony is a very small part within a larger rhythm, within a larger harmony . . That you in yourself are a very important part of a larger unit, whether this unit is your family, or your place of work, or simply the people you come in touch with throughout your life . . The more balanced, the stronger you are yourself, the more use you are as a building block, as a connecting link with everything around you . . You are like a single stitch within a knitted fabric, the importance of your life can only be assessed in relation to your connecting power between that which went before and that which is to come . .

You will find that when you look on your life in this light, it is so simplified, it becomes very much easier to be both resilient and active within your chosen or given field of activity . . Go back once more to the rhythm of your own breathing, immerse yourself, your whole being in that rhythm and all the time feel yourself expanding and relaxing more and more in all directions until you lose all sense of shape, you become like a large circle, peaceful and still and self-contained . .

Silence for twenty minutes.

Become aware of your hands and wriggle your fingers, bring awareness back to your feet and point your toes down very strongly, blink your eyes. Roll over on your left side and stretch and arch, and over on your right side and stretch and arch your body. Stand up and stretch, and feel on top of the world.

Fragments from Students'
Relaxation Experiences

I tried to collect varied expressions of the subconscious to prepare you for your own experience in Progressive Yoga Relaxation and make you familiar with the infinite variety.

I was limited in the selection as some examples were too personal and others too revealing, especially as some are still active members of the school.

All the experiences of this book are contributions from students, past and present, who consider them as helpful for beginners.

Some students kept regular diaries writing down every day's Progressive Yoga Relaxation happenings. Others chose only outstanding parts. Again others noted down only one, what they considered the most important, session. A few found it easier to express themselves in poetical form.

Three single experiences:
> Left arm at first very heavy and then becoming lighter and lighter and then floating up in the air and staying there. Wonderful feeling of dexterity.

> I am left-handed and for many years my left shoulder was very painful and limited in movement. Now it is free and unrestricted. I started to wonder if the physical arm had really risen. Will look if it ever happens again.

> As soon as I reached complete withdrawal, every muscle in my body twitched and I could not stop. After what seemed a very long time, it stopped, and I was utterly exhausted, washed out. Went to bed very early and slept

for about fifteen hours. My back pain of many years has gone.

My body is very heavy, warm and my heart is beating steadily and regularly.

It feels as though I am on a boat on a calm sea, the water lapping against the sides; the acts of inhaling and exhaling are like the waves, they gently rock me.

The rocking continues for a while and then the mood changes, and I am breathing, but as a heavy warm mass; lying there and breathing. Then the breath becomes like a mystical force which controls my rhythm. Then it changes again, I am conscious of lying on the floor, but now it is the breath of the whole world which is breathing through me. I am like a passage, the air is streaming through me, through the skin, I feel porous. I am part of the Universe, I am floating in the Universe, the air seems lighter, but yet richer and more intense. All heaviness has gone, and I have a serene feeling of belonging, I do not know to what I belong, but it does not matter, I am one with all and everything. All negative feelings leave and an overwhelming sensation of love for everything, not especially to anyone and there is only love.

After this relaxation for days on end I had a floating feeling, an absolute love for everyone and I found that whatever I did was right. Since then the strain has gone in relation to my family.

Extracts from the diaries of two students

Elena and Boris were migrants, both had university degrees in psychology, which unfortunately, were unacceptable here. They had both been through inhuman experiences during the war in different parts of Europe.

Elena had lost her husband, son and daughter in the beginning of the war and had spent many long years in displaced persons' camps. She was frail and had to depend on her salary for a living. To go back to the university would mean studying during the day, and working at night. She just did not feel strong enough to do it. She was employed as a nurse in a mental hospital and felt completely lost and without an aim in life. Boris was a male nurse at the same institution and wanted to marry her, but Elena was not so sure that she wanted to remarry.

Boris was a divorcee, who had married in haste shortly after arriving here. His wife, an Australian, had left him soon after the marriage. He was tall, broad and very strong, and like a lot of Eastern European men, he felt superior to women. He had no desire to repeat his degree and felt that his qualifications were better than the equivalent here.

I suggested relaxation to them, and they did it together. I realised Boris only consented to please Elena. The first few sessions in the school had virtually no effect on them. They could not settle down and, also, had a certain resentment to my Swiss-German accent. After a few sessions at the school, and at home, they had practically decided to give up; then the reaction came.

They kept a diary of their recollections after relaxation for me:

> Elena: Have become used to M.S.'s accent for the first time.
> Feeling of withdrawal. Sinking sensation, slowly sinking
> downwards. Pleasant sensation.

> Boris: Legs and arms quickly very heavy, then the whole
> body. After a while the body felt one big mass of indefinite
> shape.

> Elena: Saw plants, all sorts of arrangements of plants.
> Especially the stems, where the leaves grow, in all the
> different ways, at regular intervals, irregular intervals,
> opposite each other, and spiralling up the stem. It was
> beautiful and calming. I was reluctant to come back to
> full consciousness.

> Boris: Felt as though I was floating, and being aware of
> two parts of myself, one lying and one floating. Knew
> they were both me, did not like to go and put the floating
> part back into the lying body. Lost consciousness, and
> got quite a shock when M.S. started talking again.

> Elena: Very pleasant, again the sensation of sinking deeper,
> this time an all-embracing warmth. Feeling very warm
> in the back of the head, in the cerebellum. Felt very good
> all day. My brain was completely free from worry, felt
> very active and brighter than usual.

Boris: Felt very easy and warm in the chest, sheltered, protected feeling, several times lost voice.

Elena: My eyes were very tense and it took a while to relax and lose the feeling of tension, started thinking what it could mean, then sank again very deep and had a blissful feeling of complete peace of mind. Would have liked to continue.

Boris: Saw latch with key dropped out of door. All tests I could challenge, but it was more of a struggle than to follow suggestions. Felt very fresh after session.

Elena: The knowledge of each coming word gave me deep peace and a feeling of security. Instantaneously went into deep relaxation. Didn't hear much. Was practically all the time in my inner consciousness.

Boris: Throughout the session a feeling of peace and light.

Elena: Felt rather agitated, and frustrated, slowly the voice induced relaxation. Went very deep, saw a big tree, saw above the earth the beautiful foliage, and in the earth lovely roots. Feeling the strength and being very secure. Felt like being the tree and having very deep roots. Afterwards felt strong and serene, and for the first time completely at home in Australia.

Boris: Started the session with toothache and in a bad mood, shortly after was in a deep sleep. The toothache disappeared only a slight residue of feeling in that spot persists. Bad temper gone.

Elena: Saw the cells splitting in two and going on, and one cell having a pulse and developing. The cells were very clear and in beautiful colours. All the centres going together and like an hour-glass — dividing into yet more cells.

Boris: Went very deep then saw coloured stripes going past. Then all the colours together, as in a rainbow. Felt very uplifted and light.

Elena: It was a dark night, very rough sea. Was bouncing up and down in the sea. Felt exhausted and at the point of drowning. Wanted something to hold on to, finally found a rock I could hold on to, then it was less dark, and a larger rock came into sight, then a rocky shore,

I collapsed exhausted and half conscious. After a while sitting up and looking towards the water, I saw many people struggling in the water, who were desperately in need of help. By holding on to one of the rocks, I succeeded in helping one person out, then helped a few more. When they had recovered, we made a human chain to help more and more to safety. We worked till all were saved and we all sat on the rocky shore.

Boris: Very quickly reached the borderline of sleep. This state getting deeper and deeper. After a while the body feels more sleepy and mental state seems to be much clearer. I had a couple of visions.
The first: Cleansing a vessel, my wife used for watering the garden. I immersed this one in the sea.
The second: From the bridge a man brought back a small boy who went astray far away to the left. Feeling man and the boy are one and the same person.

Elena: Went immediately very deep, only feeling was one of contentment, and without desire.

Boris: At the beginning, I saw a symbol of waking state in the mind's eye. There are two directions of mental energy, one projecting outwards, the other whirling around like a mill, in the middle of the brain. Saw it clearly turning in the brain and the other going out through my head into the world.

Elena: I stand on a needle-like rock. There is just enough room to stand comfortably. All sides fall vertically down many hundred metres. I am completely at ease and unafraid. My fear of heights has vanished, and I enjoy the beautiful view, turning slowly around to take it all in. Then a strong wind starts to blow, it does not affect me. I stand solid like a rock and the wind blowing through me gives me a feeling of newness.

Boris: At first glimpses from the memory about the physical world. Then attention inside my body; still fragments of the physical world. As in a dream some pictures came forward, and everything else was lost.

Elena: It feels as if my shoulders expand and become very large. Something flows from the shoulders and neck forward to the chest. I am not quite sure if it flows through the chest or around it, but even the shoulders flow downwards. The neck is warm and heavy, a warm and heavy mass is flowing down from the shoulders and neck into the middle of the body. This heavy mass continues to flow forward, out of the chest and like very pleasant warm water down over the body.

Boris: Several seconds and already some memory pictures start to appear. Pictures like in dreams came shortly afterwards. I hear the word 'lightness' and see a car with wings floating through the air. I see the picture of a small child (new-born?). New patient or new type of suggestion to be used, it is very hard to interpret symbols. The pictures change very quickly. From time to time I hear the voice but not the words. I did not feel the body, but was very much aware of my ego. The physical world disappeared, I was like in a dream.

Elena: I felt like an underwater plant and swayed gently with the water. Afterwards I realised that the swaying was in accord with the rhythm of the breath. The water was flowing through me as well as around me and the sea creatures swam and moved around me, oblivious of my presence. I am just part of the sea — I just am and belong here.

Boris: Stiffening of the face muscles. After a while, relaxing part after part and then losing M.S.'s voice. There is no projection of mental energy. There is no struggle of forces. After that lost the voice most of the time. Afterwards felt refreshed, rested and alert.

Elena: After the last session felt the lightness of the water plant for many days. My work was much easier — was not at all tired. Tried to recreate the same experience — unsuccessfully — gave up and relaxed very deeply. The breathing became conscious with a delightful rhythm. A pleasant feeling of warmth penetrates with the rhythm in every cell inducing a kind of bubbly feeling. I have the sensation of complete cleansing of everything in me.

Boris: A couple of pains in different parts of the body. Deeply relaxed especially the nerves. Made the decision to think about something else. But after a while I realised the pictures coming into my mind were following the suggestions.

103

Elena had not only become much stronger during the past year, but there was a wonderful quality of being alive about her. She had taken charge of a rather old-fashioned home for mentally retarded children, modernised and generally improved it. Her approach to the children was remarkable — music, dancing, painting, modelling clay; love, patience and kindness were her medium to teach and what had once been a rather depressing and drab institution was now a happy colourful place.

Her enthusiasm inspired a group of active young matrons to help individually with a roster system and also financially as a group by way of sales, collections, luncheon parties and lectures.

Boris left the school after Elena had gone interstate. He did not choose to discuss his future with me so I do not know where he is, but he did become easier to get on with, more humane.

Excerpts from the diary of an agnostic who found faith

Had an extremely pleasant session of Progressive Yoga Relaxation. After a fairly long period of restless eyes, they suddenly quietened down to a wonderful 'standstill' and 'silence'; no visual disturbances.

It takes me at least ten minutes until my eyes quieten, then there will be a fairly even nothingness; but thoughts intrude easily and the slightest motion of the eyes produces a pattern which makes me feel that the patterns I see are physiological consequence. On the other hand, I feel certain that it would only be during complete oblivion and nothingness that I could comprehend that 'otherness' for which we have no word symbol. And this 'otherness' must not be of a 'god-like' nature in the generally accepted sense of God, but of cosmic nature.

Finished reading *Worlds in Collision;* for a very long time have not been impressed by a book as by this one. I am not a scientist, therefore cannot blow holes in it with scientific arguments; to me it is so logical that Velikovsky's theory could just be right and not mere theory. He certainly has helped channel my thoughts towards my cosmic views.

104

Cannot say anything novel about my experience in Progressive Yoga Relaxation. As a matter of fact I find the mere expectance of some possible happening is a hindrance to letting go.

Have been to one lesson at night, although I enjoyed Progressive Yoga Relaxation, I cannot enjoy it as much as when alone with M.S.

I am sleeping well as always after period. I am also not as harassed at work. I am still at cross-purposes with my own self as to what to do, which way I want to go concerning a profession. Continue to drift like a coward, hoping that something will decide for me. As to my private life, I know I am tied. To run away from it cannot be done with a good conscience, so I want to take it with the equanimity I always pray for.

Had the second Progressive Yoga Relaxation in the school. M.S. was very kind and addressed herself to me, I felt, by being silent longer than usual. Body was soon senseless, non-existent. In spite of noises (wind, door opening, man next to me snoring gently) they registered, but did not disturb or upset. Mind was restive and yet alert. Saliva had stopped. The after-effects are always pleasant, because of the all-pervading quietude of mind. I am still extremely tired and I decided to concentrate on the following four:

> Health and strength.
> Materially, to do the right and correct thing at all times, in all my actions which should bring me to decisions regarding my future. Intellectually, to be permitted to take active part in stage direction in amateur theatre. Spiritually, to fulfil myself, to find union with the cosmic, universal force.

Have not written for a long time as everything proceeded unchanged. My greatest trouble is obviously that I expect a change or just expect something to happen, without any decision on my part. This is probably my greatest fault. I am on a week's leave and enjoy the freedom; I am very tired and hope that few days' rest will help. Last session with M.S. was a little more successful.

That week's holiday was one of the hardest of my life, trying to battle out things with myself. Could not come to terms with anything, felt very depressed, frustrated, and utterly lost. Only towards the end of the week did I seem to get some sort of zest for life. Saw Dr. R. on Friday. All is well physically. He helped me by telling me that my part in life is to find peace within myself despite the conditions immediately around me.

At M.S. I felt deep peace and approached a condition of deep-blue to light-blue blissful nothingness.

Months have passed since my last entry. A lot has happened, yet nothing.

Have had upsetting weeks and months. Summer very hot and disturbing. Two bad colds after each other in spite of injections. Holiday enjoyable, but too short. Have not been to the school since November, but had many talks with M.S. She is showing a surprising interest in me for which I am grateful. During our talks I benefit more from her teaching than class. My relaxations have been most unsatisfactory. Twenty minutes is really not enough. Must try to have more time.

Have read two books which impressed me very much because they stress what I have vaguely felt for a long time; that Christ's teachings are metaphysical ones, of a high degree, put into garbled everyday language to make it gullible for the great masses. God is the benevolent father with a kindly face and long beard only in those fable-like biblical accounts because the great abstraction of Universal Power — Universal Mind, and its complete neutrality towards everything, is too hard to grasp and, for most, too unappealing.

I had a very bad weekend with a cold which has developed into an unpleasant nasal catarrh. I took some pills which are effective but leave me limp, hot and muggy.

How difficult it is to abstract oneself from thinking habits one has been accustomed to for a lifetime — to ban such thoughts as 'I hope I won't catch a cold', 'I hope the cold won't get worse,' etc. which are so difficult to suppress. I realise and understand the negativity and harmfulness of such thinking, but I do not know how to actively put into operation what, in theory, I understand. On the whole there is so much I understand, I do accept ideas as correct in my reading, but I cannot apply them in practice. If I could get some more guidance in practical work. The main thing would be to have peaceful and quiet surroundings for much longer each day, not just ten to fifteen minutes daily for relaxation. Only in silence can one's soul grow and come to grips with the un-nameable; of that I am sure. But where to get this peace and silence from in this restless era of ours? Perhaps it is my life's task to achieve my inner peace in spite of the noise, haste, and jarring of nerves.

It has been clear to me for a long time that mind is what matters most, that is the determining factor of one's whole make-up, the be-all and end-all of the condition of one's existence.

Consequently, as long as I continue to harbour such vague ideas about my future plans, or rather, no-plans at all, I shall continue to flounder and nothing definite is ever bound to happen unless I shall will it so.

S.A.

In making this selection from the student diary-notes for the purpose of the present book two aspects were considered. I intentionally left out those notes written in a positive and confident frame of mind which mingled with the others in order to demonstrate with emphasis the exceeding despondency and negativeness which came to the surface as a result of the cleansing effect of the relaxation practised by the student, who, to the outside world seemed calm, collected, unruffled, cheerful. This, no doubt, was due to self-discipline.

The second aspect governing my choice from the notes was to stress the time factor. The work done and the results achieved stretched not just over months, but years, and continued after the date when the diary notes ended. Although not inevitably so, cleansing through relaxation is not a swift affair; circumstances and the sincerity of effort amongst others playing a vital part.

The student continued to work even if no further notes were taken and persists in daily sessions of either relaxation or meditation. The almost painful expression in the existing notes of the constant and paralysing fatigue, the indecision, aimlessness and sense of futility simmered like some unholy threat, underground, gathering strength only to be hurled out like so much debris by a later illness, not unlike a volcano erupting once the inner force became powerful enough to catapult the boiling matter sky-high.

Relieved by the impact of that catharsis and genuinely calmed, the student's attitude to life changed extensively. There was a sudden understanding and seeing of the self, which ushered in a period of peace of mind and a contentment in a new search, inward this time, striving to place this inner self into its proper perspective or relationship to that Cosmic Plan suggested in the notes. This inner calm soon started to reflect in physical health, a well-balanced body, and a kind of lovely radiance, and the deadly tiredness vanished. Acceptance of any situation through understanding took over from the earlier rebellion and discontent. But, above all, the awareness that no matter what kind of situation needs to be experienced or faced, it is for the benefit of the person concerned, has given the student an ease in living which has paved the way to a balanced life in which joy is deeply felt and adversity does not upset.

> Every experience
> Every encounter
> In the last instance
> A form of learning.
>
> Each day's struggle
> Each joy and sorrow
> Fragmented wisdom
> Laboriously gathered
>
> Of this collection
> Lovingly offered
> Can help our brother
> In times of need
>
> Then all experience
> And all encounters
> Have served their purpose
> Fulfilled their aim.

> B.M.

The following notes were recorded in diary sequence by Sarah as they occurred over a twenty-one week period:

On the voyage to Australia, I was then approximately eight, my father, after a quarrel with my mother, disappeared. I searched all over the ship, and as time passed and I could not find him, I was afraid he had jumped overboard.

When I was about four or five a pig was to be slaughtered on a neighbouring farm. For weeks the children discussed the coming feast with mounting excitement in which I was fully included. They pointed out a hook fastened low in a wall, which played some part in holding the pig while the farmer killed it. On the actual day, after the parts for curing, etc. were put aside, all the bits and pieces and organs were boiled and cooked in enormous pots to be eaten at the 'Schlachfest'. The farmer's large family and friends all joined in this gorging with pig's meat.

Afterwards my parents fully explained to me about Jews not being permitted to eat pork.

We lived in Altenburg now and I was about six. A neighbour sent me to her butcher on a message. It was the custom to ask a child from which sausage it would like a hunk.

The lady asked me to choose, but I told her I wasn't allowed, because it wasn't kosher. She poo-poohed this and told me, kindly, she wouldn't tell anyone, to go ahead and eat it. I walked out without it, but how I hungered after that sausage.

Scared still of falling out of upper bunk during voyage to Australia.

Watching parade of Nazi might.

Children in village took me with them to Church where I knelt and prayed to Virgin Mary. I think it was Easter.

Jerking of limbs.

Saw pictures of a lake. At the same time the thought: 'I haven't seen this before'. Then I lost consciousness. Upon being aware again the thought: 'This time I relaxed more deeply than for a long time past.'

In a railway waiting room, after a trip to Poland by my mother and myself, she discovered that my hair was crawling with lice. Though she took all possible action to rid me of them I remained terrified that when I went back to school in a few days the health inspector might still discover something in my hair. A girl in my class had had to have her hair shaved and wore a woollen cap for a long time. The whole school knew about her and she was virtually an outcast.

When breathing in and out felt as though breathing in love and breathing out love.

A band of flames across the horizon advances towards me. As it lies on the ground my body burns.

I had a dream in which my mother was well until I poisoned her and she died. The murder was not discovered. The months after the funeral I lived in constant dread and guilt. In the instant of coming out of the dream I found I was questioning myself. Where had I bought the poison tablets? How had I administered them? Doubt and hope entered my mind when I could not answer. By this time I was aware of my husband next to me in bed. He spoke, but I did not answer. I had to find out for sure whether I was guilty or not. I felt frightfully guilty.

Only very slowly the real facts of my mother's illness came back to me. I didn't know whether to believe them or not. I had to back them up with recollections of her years in and out of hospitals, of the doctor telling us she had cancer. In the dream I had remembered nothing of this. It was some time after I was half awake that I understood clearly that I was not a murderer; that I had not poisoned her.

First, I saw a globe and shade, then repeated for the rest of the hour: 'Turn off the light', just as I had heard my father say it to me thousands of times.

Remembered my loneliness when at the age of about five, we shifted from Kohren to the small town of Altenburg. I missed my former, constant companion, Renate. I became ill with fever. Towards the close of the relaxation, and until its end, I repeated in my mind — 'Renate, Renate, Renate'.

One evening when I was four or five my parents left the house for a while. Awakened from sleep by knocking at the window of my bedroom I heard a man's voice talking into my room.

I screamed, 'Go away! Go away!' until he left.

At last my parents returned and, beside myself, I told them of my terror. To my astonishment they did not believe me. My mother maintained it must have been a nightmare. My father conceded finally that 'someone may have played a joke', then I kept yelling, 'No it happened, it happened!'

Long afterwards a farm-labourer from another village told my father he had come to see him one evening. Finding the place in unexpected darkness he had knocked on the side bedroom window hoping the child would tell him where her parents were. When the child did not listen to him, but kept on yelling, he returned to his village.

My body was destroyed by a great furry animal down to the skeleton. Then, in one instant, it became restored.

A few months after our arrival in Australia, when I was ten, there occurred a frightful quarrel between my parents. For the first time there was a threat of violence. In my fearful apprehension I prayed to God to prevent this imminent catastrophe and I would give up all claims to future happiness.

All important was that the dreadful thing about to occur be prevented. In return God should deny me anything I desired from now on.

I bent backwards, my body growing until the earth, meanwhile shrinking into a smaller globe, was encircled by my stretched limbs.

At seventeen I was in an agony of under-the-surface apprehension. What could I do when my mother shifted from our flat into a house she was buying in which to live with the Soldier husband she had recently married? He was the most kind-hearted of men, but I knew I could never live there with them.

From out of the darkness under a bridge a man in a rowing boat, his body and head wound about with bandages, finds his path blocked by an iron grille. Dropping the oars, with his bare hands, exerting his whole strength, he bends back the ironwork until he has made a gap large enough for him to pass through.

The bandages disappear. He rows on.

A door with key in lock, attached to key is a ring from which hangs more keys.

There welled from the region of my heart and solar plexus, as though from a spring, an intensity of feeling much as I have not known before.

111

Uncountable golden spheres floated in this living flood of feeling, spreading continually outwards.

I don't know if it lasted five minutes, ten minutes, or a quarter of an hour. In the instant when I realised it was fading there was such a contrast between what had gone before and ordinary reality again, which seemed so dull and flat by comparison, that I tried to cling on. But the very fact of thinking, meant, of course that it was gone.

For days afterwards I felt thrilled and happy.

The many, many hours of mental exercises were immeasurably worth those few minutes.

These experiences were helping Sarah to make a major decision without the slightest doubt. During training for a swimming competition her son collapsed and was rushed to the nearest hospital. After a few days he was transferred to the renal unit for special tests. The results of these tests were disastrous. Both kidneys were shrunk and in an acute state of infection, beyond recovery leaving only one possibility, removal of the damaged organs and a transplant.

Initially, the patient was too sick for any major treatment and before the operation he had to be on the dialysis machine for artificial blood cleansing. Sebastian revolted against the use of the kidney machine as he had heard terrible things about its dulling effect of the mind from other patients. His doctor put this right and his mother explained to him the necessity of acceptance from the esoteric point of view.

The human being is goal-orientated. This applies to both body and mind. Part of that success-mindedness also includes a wonderful defence mechanism, the ability to reject infections and foreign cells of any kind. The subconscious cannot distinguish between unwanted and wanted cells, for instance a transplant, and the body rejects it. This is the reason why transplants are still so difficult in spite of the extremely high surgical standard. The patient can help with not being antagonistic, or even better, with actual desire and to welcome the treatment thereby influencing the defence system to accept the new cells. This also applies to the artificial cleansing of the blood through the dialysis machine.

Sebastian was eager to try out anything which would improve his condition. He applied pranayama, yoga relaxation and suggestions. After some weeks he was ready to be connected to the machine for several days each week. Sebastian, by the way, was the only patient who did not get sick when he was joined to the machine for the first time. This made a tremendous impression on him and it gave him the necessary impetus to concentrate even harder on his mental programme.

Unknown to anyone, Sarah, his mother, underwent all the tests to become a live donor. Most transplants come from dead bodies, as there are very few people emotionally ready for such a sacrifice. The experiences with live donors show that afterwards they are inclined to have difficulty in adjusting psychologically. Some never quite overcome the mental shock and are handicapped for the rest of their lives. A donor must not reason himself into doing it, his decision must be spontaneous. His whole being has to accept unconditionally the idea of giving a vital part of his own body away and there must not be the slightest doubt or any uneasiness about it. There is an enormous psychological difference between deciding to have a healthy organ cut out of the body or to have a life-endangering sick part removed to save one's life. The goal-orientated subconscious revolts against the sacrifice of a healthy part and has to be specially prepared by the individual himself.

For the transplant to be successful the organ has to be from a similar type. For instance an identical twin is perfect. Brother or sister would rate second best. Mother and father each have half of the necessary points. There also exists total strangers with enough affinity to be used as a donor.

Sebastian had to wait again a few weeks after the removal of his kidneys till he was strong enough for the transplant. It was an outstanding success and as it was the first live transplant to be done at this hospital, the surgical team, Sebastian and Sarah were in the news for a day or two.

It is nearly two years now; both are very well and Sebastian will do his matriculation this year.

Diary of a woman with too great an attachment to her children, relatives and friends, who mostly took advantage of her affection, leaving her in a perpetual state of exhaustion and frustration. She is now a very contented individual coping efficiently and discriminately with the different demands on her time and person.

I am looking downwards and see two meat hooks, one each side, embedded in my exposed brain. With slow, careful hands I disengage the hooks from the soft mass. The hooks are rusty and look as though they have been lodged there for a long time, but when they are removed the brain closes up and is neither scarred nor damaged.

The inner ear hears what is inaudible to the outer ear. With the mind's eye one sees what is invisible to the eye. If the senses have these subtler states, there must also be a subtler state of the mind, a mind's mind, an inner mind that is not dependent on interpretation of the senses, however subtle. I would like to know this mind.

For some moments the feeling of protective waves emanating outwards a few feet past my body. Could not resist trying to recapture it, but the only result was a sense of strain.

Had hallucinations as though I watched my body, which was in a horizontal position, moving upwards, becoming smaller in the distance, till it merged into the sun.

Suddenly it seems as though my legs were being stretched and there was a tremendous pull between foot soles and crown. It could be compared to the tension and pull in elastic, which fixed at one end, is stretched from the other.

Standing on its own, without a background, a large tree its branches thick with leaves and rounded in outline is suddenly transformed into a stark signpost pointing in four directions. But there is no writing on the pointers.

To go to the Yoga School one had to climb a not quite perpendicular wall of dark-grey, rough-hewn square stones. The stones, rigid in their places, provided an abundance of hand and footholds.

One day I became aware of a change. Here and there I found loose stones, so to avoid disaster I had to examine each stone carefully.

Then came the last trip. A very fat woman, younger than I, climbed with me. There were no secure stones any more. Every one rolled, the more so the higher I climbed. I became consumed by fear. The only way I avoided crashing down with one of the loose stones was extremely careful compensatory placing of my weight.

The fat girl urged me to hurry, complaining that I was retarding her progress by my slowness. She jeered at my groping to test a stone, the last one, upon which I must place both my feet and my whole weight, before pulling myself over the rim to the top. Instinct warned me not to listen to her, to rely on myself. It was the trickiest stone of all and I took infinite care in balancing myself.

At the top, when I looked down, to my utter surprise I saw that there was a road leading to the top: a wide, smooth, gently graded bitumen highway that I could henceforth take.

The emotions of this experience were particularly vivid and for hours afterwards I felt the fear still in the pit of the stomach.

I have a rope ring around my neck from which branch ropes as in a maypole, the ends of which are held by various people. The slightest tug results in pressure on my neck. I am forced to respond to the pull. I am nearly driven mad by the tugging of these people, but to survive I must go in whatever direction I am pulled.

Then I cut the rope-ring around my neck, and as I see the whole maypole collapse and the people now powerless to move me, I am absolutely amazed that one such simple action, one cut, was sufficient to free me.

Thick iron chain. Axe falls from above and cuts it in two.

The innermost is the same in everyone. The core of the earth is the same for the mountain, the desert and the sea.

The thought, just as physical stones can form in the gall-bladder and can be removed, so mental stones can form and can be removed.

Then saw myself standing at a crater-like opening. A stone detached itself from me and dropped into water which was so far down that I saw the splash but could not hear it.

Saw a thick dark brown layer peel itself off me. The skin underneath was clean and fresh.

Became aware that I am connected to people by thick, artery-like attachments issuing from my solar-plexus to theirs. It seems to make no difference whether the people are living or dead or whether I am in daily contact with them or have not seen them for years.

If a situation occurred with an emotion, positive or negative, the pulsating cord-like attachment was there.

115

To get free I held an oxywelding torch which I used backwards and forwards on the cord till it appeared blackened and charred and dropped off, or simply disintegrated and disappeared. This I did as many times as I became consciously aware of it.

A pair of scales, between earth and the sky. I sit in one dish, the other is empty. I throw parts of myself over into the other dish. Not physical parts, attributes rather. As the dish on the other side becomes heavier and goes down, I go up. After a while I go down again and the whole process is repeated again and again.

After each repetition the whole set of scales moves a fraction upwards.

Realised that the immensity of the solar system and all space in between are one entity, in the same way as the separate parts of a human being make up one entity.

The sun was about to set beyond the horizon. Desire never to let the sun out of my sight. Was able to travel so fast over the surface of the earth that I never lost sight of it. It was immensely satisfying to have the sun always before me.

Felt that gravity is the love of earth for everything on it.
Felt part of a group, but as an individual.

The etheric body is used by will to transmit to physical body.

G.R.

Spiral.

Guard: when mine were your cruel eyes
There was music in the arena
And applause from the citizens,
Their suffering is visited upon me in another age
which hides its victims in unspeakable places
But the Law is unchanged.

When the tiger stamped on the graves
                                    the dead appeared.
Where is the gondolier to take us there?
Give us a rope to climb there!
The clamour was awful for none knew the way.
They stank in their fear.
Do not leave us in our bodies!
He bared his teeth to rend them.
Is it necessary? They wailed,
It is necessary.

G.R.

Wings of Power

Up to the present time, mankind has made very little use of the power of the mind. In fact, we have only just scratched its surface. But now that we have entered the new age of Aquarius, man will advance at a hitherto undreamed of rate.

Nothing in the Universe is possible without first being created in the mind. Take any invention, no matter how small or how large; something insignificant such as a change of programme on the spur of the moment, or the mending of some object in an unorthodox manner; take any creation from a satellite to a new household gadget — everything has first to be thought of. First there has to be a desire, a mental picture, a sort of blueprint; then a mould into which unmanifest matter — ether — can flow to cast the creation. This can take from a few minutes to many years and involve many different minds. The more thought that goes into a project, the more complex will be the result.

If thoughts dwell long enough, and with enough concentration, on the same subject, the channel is built for an inrush from the Universal Mind's storage of ether. Every individual amongst us can do it; the only requirement is a good idea and concentration held long enough to contact the Universal Mind so that the inflow can take place. This can be used for anything, whether it be spiritual, physical, philosophical, scientific, business, or a problem in our daily life.

Every thought which has ever been thought stays in the Universe. The clearer, more precise and the more accurately formulated it is, the more it will be impressed on the Universal Mind as nothing is ever lost. Every thought belongs to a certain wave-length. As soon as a person thinks along that wave-length, the already existing ideas of that wave-length are available to the 'tuned-in' thinker. This is one of the reasons why in different corners of the world, similar ideas are conceived and created. This applies not only to complicated scientific inventions, but to simple things in daily life. There is what the German language defines as 'Zeitgeist', meaning the spirit of the times or the drift of thought and feeling in a period, a tendency to think similar thoughts, to be concerned about the same ideas; and is symptomatic of every epoch.

The most advanced beings of each and every age catch up with the current trends of the time and develop an idea even further, taking conscious or unconscious advantage of the already existing thought forms of the times and of the Universal Mind. Very few people are conscious of this; as a rule man is unaware of the source of his ideas.

Some sensory type people think wonderful, very advanced thoughts, but do not put them into practice; they are quite happy just to think of them. But, as the Universal Mind stores their thoughts, the next person thinking along these lines, and applying them concretely, will benefit by all of these previously conceived ideas. No thought is ever lost in the Universe. How often do we marvel when a person brings forth ideas which appear to be above his ability? It is work and application which account for this. Even the very highest I.Q. is lost when not used properly, whereas a not so high standard of intelligence, continuously and assiduously applied to the task at hand, can have astonishing results through the law of attraction.

A philosophy professor, an old friend of mine, used to say: 'I prefer at any time a student who is dedicated to his work, to a lazy genius.' Whilst I do not fully agree with this remark, as there are certain conclusions and inventions which can only be arrived at by a genius, there is a lot to be said for a disciplined, concentrated application by a lesser-endowed mind.

Women are more sensitive to the 'Zeitgeist', but as passivity is the female attribute, they are not always in a position where they can use this gift of sensitivity.

In our time total equality between man and woman will come about. Woman will, at last, be given the same status as man. By this I do not mean that she will do everything in a manly way; on the contrary she will be different from him, she will be herself and please herself, as man now pleases himself. A woman who tries to copy man still makes herself servile, but in a different way. Up to this time, the female, being predominantly passive by nature was rarely given the chance to venture into the abstract, as this was mainly male territory. As with all changes there is at first exaggeration; the pendulum swinging too far to the other side, as is shown in some aspects of women's lib. That movement is absolutely necessary. Without aggression change is much too slow.

This active and passive reaction does not only apply to the human race, but to all living organisms; and even to all things positive and negative. These laws apply to the whole Universe, to the Macrocosmos as well as to the Microcosmos. The more one realises this, the more one becomes awed about the Creator of all. We can only grasp the tiniest bit of the greatness of the Universe and its creatures, and apply the knowledge to gain more wisdom. The only way to prove our understanding of the Universal Laws is to live them. This will make the human being ready to tap the Universal Mind for its glorious ideas.

The human being is the highest on Earth — not in the Universe — there are more evolved beings on other planets. The human race is a chosen one, that is why we have so much free will.

We have a rhythm, caused by our metabolism, soul, temperament and inheritance. Positive and negative, or active and passive, should be balanced. Feeling things, listening to music, television, or any other viewing, collecting, automatic work, are all passive. To create, to do new things, having to think as you work, are active. Most people do more passive living and so their active impulses are not used enough for creation, but that impulse is still there showing itself as aggression. We must balance these two forces so that we can make the most of our life.

With every single thought, a human being has to decide whether it is to be positive or negative. Let's start with the morning, do we open our eyes immediately or a little later? Every action has to be decided, we are always torn between two ways, positive or negative. Never are we allowed to take it easy in this respect, if we do, Karma takes care that we learn our lesson.

The human being has the knowledge of good and evil, and the potential sense of discrimination — to know when to be silent and when to talk; to know when to love and when to be indifferent. These opposites are:

Love	Indifferent
Loyalty	Non-attachment
Love of life	Contempt of death
Courage	Caution
To rule	To serve
To talk	To be silent
Confidence	Humility
Prudence	Quick action
Acceptance	Discrimination
Peace	Ability to fight
Receptivity	Resistance to influence
To own the whole world	To have no possessions

All forces of nature are neutral. Man, in using them, changes them into positive or negative powers. We are here on this earth to learn to use these forces in the right way. To use the right force at the right moment makes us evolved beings, conscious co-workers of the Universe.

We must apply our free will in everything we do as we have approximately three-quarters Karma — compulsion and one-quarter free will. Our free will of today creates our Karma of tomorrow. In fact Karma is possible only through free will. Because of the free will we can decide our emotional moods every second of our lives, each mood producing an equivalent vibration. The law of attraction and repulsion applies not only to chemistry, but to the whole Universe. Whatever vibration you send out, the equivalent wave-length will return to you.

The thoughts you think have their own vibrations — wavelengths. If you are full of compassion, with every breath Prana (life-force) nourishes this emotion and the same wavelength will come rushing in.

The free will should also be used in thought control, during the day when there is compulsory association. Now these associated thoughts have nothing whatsoever to do with the conscious mind, intelligence or free will. The subconscious is allowed to react as it pleases. There are a great number of people, who do not think one original thought for weeks on end, and fewer still who apply it after having thought it. The average person is, most of the time, quite unconscious of his thoughts and only very few would be able to account for their day and what they thought, say for the preceding seventeen hours. The more the subconscious is in charge during the day, the greater the working during sleep (REM) to shed all these trivial, unnecessary and harmful thoughts.

We have forgotten how to be still in ourself. We allow the mind to race ahead, always thinking ahead, planning ahead, concerned only about the future, forgetting that we can only live and appreciate the present. It is the present which counts, as we can only be truly conscious of the present, provided we apply ourselves to it. If the work you do is very mechanical, then you should keep your mind still and enjoy the present; if after a while your mind starts wandering, and you are in a situation which permits you to recite or sing, then do so, otherwise repeat a mantram silently. It is simply a matter of avoiding indulging in trivial useless little thoughts, because they can be very destructive.

If people were only aware of the harm they do by filling themselves up to overflowing with unimportant, and most of the time negative, thoughts they would avoid them. The uncontrolled mind endlessly repeats offences against itself, or resorts to argument, going over and over the details and giving the answers missed in the heat of the argument. Then people wonder why they quarrel, and say hurtful and cruel things to each other, maintaining afterwards that they didn't have such thoughts before and feeling quite bewildered. The truth is, whatever you think will have to come out of you in some way. It is like this, if you fill a bottle with clear water, only clear water will come out of it; fill it with ink and ink will come out of it. A computer can only answer questions connected with its own data. Consequently, out of a person comes only that which the person thinks (puts in).

If meditation does not fit easily into your western way of living; Karma Yoga would then be best suited to the average western way of life. This yoga of right action transforms everything done into an act of awareness, all physical work becomes a means of learning one's lesson in this world. The very work of one's hands undergoes a metamorphosis into higher consciousness. Most western people consider eastern teaching to be fit only for the inactive dreamer, who, away from the busy world lives in seclusion — meditating. The way of the yogi who goes into seclusion is rather the exception, most of the eastern people follow the path of Karma Yoga. The Karma yogi has to understand that he is just a tiny, but useful part of the overall plan of life. He has to fulfil his part, be content with complete devotion, without anxiety. Some western people would always like to jump ahead, to hasten their advancement. They cannot understand why everything has to move so slowly and not only just slowly, but that there has to be a constant repetition of similar episodes and happenings. We have to go through each experience in life on many occasions until it is burned into our soul. Only then will we stop reacting wrongly, then we will rather give up life than deny the truth.

For this same reason all situations and circumstances have to be experienced personally. No one can experience them for another being. To be told of an experience is understanding it on the intellectual level and is only the very earliest beginning. Only what we have emotionally experienced ourselves, what we have felt in our own heart, will make an impression on our soul, and only a very deep impression will last forever. That is why we learn exclusively through suffering, deepest suffering which keeps us awake, makes us ask for help in sleepless nights, when we are lost in darkness and there seems to be no way out. When we reach the point of desperation, when we feel we can't continue any more, when we stop blaming others for our troubles and when we slowly and reluctantly admit our faults and shortcomings to ourselves — then we will have solved that special problem.

We have to experience all suffering so many times that under no circumstances would we be capable of inflicting such pain onto another being again. Some people think we should have remained in the primitive state of our early forefathers, who, in actual fact, were more balanced than we are now. They had reached this balance on the instinctive level. Our aim is to reach it on the conscious level. We are meant to purposely do the right thing at all times, so that to hurt will no longer be possible to our nature. This should not only apply to our deeds and acts, but also to our thoughts.

Stillness is a state of mind and one does not need to sit in meditation for it. We can achieve it on a solitary walk, at work, actually anywhere; we should be perceptive and not allow our thoughts to race around. To work and have the next task race ahead in the mind is even worse. To be hours ahead has a devastating effect on our subconscious sense of time. Let me put it this way: The instinctive mind is reached through emotion and the strongest emotion will win through. For instance, a job is done rather mechanically, which means unemotionally; simultaneously the mind is intensely, that is emotionally, occupied with a job two hours hence.

Therefore, for the subconscious it is already that time, and the two hours in between are as good as lost. Because of this, no matter how much this person tries to accomplish, he will always be short of time, as he loses precious hours every day through this racing ahead.

If you want practically unlimited time for all you would like to do, stop your mind from racing ahead, plan your day with concentration. You can always save time by planning a timetable, by jotting down your plans; it will take only a few minutes. Then strive to still your mind, instead of jumping ahead.

There is a type of brainwashing which happens when people are critical and often think of others in a disapproving manner. Take for example; a young married woman who starts her new way of life full of enthusiasm and good will. After the first few months have passed, settling into her daily routine, she starts to notice a few shortcomings in her husband. Perhaps he was used to his mother putting his clothes away, therefore he is rather untidy. The young wife criticises him in her mind, especially if, even after asking him to be more orderly, he forgets. Over the years, if the young woman is not conscious of it, her criticism will sharpen, she will think less lovingly of him and his attributes and more of his faults. If she does not realise this and check it in time, she will systematically brainwash herself out of love.

This naturally also applies to a man who can in time brainwash himself out of love with his wife, for some similar reasons. You cannot feed all of these negative thoughts to your subconscious without them lashing out from time to time. It is in instances such as this that people say awful things to each other in anger. They are themselves shocked and will say later: 'But, I did not mean it, I do not know what came over me, how could I say things I don't even think.' The fact is they do think them, only they do not realise it. The subconscious has to be treated with respect and not as a garbage bin. Remember, it is only that which is put in, which will come out.

Most worries come from having to make decisions. The greatest strain on a mind is indecision, weighing and pondering over a problem until utterly confused. During sleepless nights the simplest problem will take on gigantic proportions, until all sense of value is lost.

Exhausted after a night battling worries, one is not able to understand what actually happened, why the problem was insoluble, when in the morning it does not seem so bad. One should never think about problems before going to sleep, this is the wrong time.

The sun's characteristics are positive, creative, extrovert, piercing straight forward, without deviation, whereas the moon is negative, sustaining, introvert, building a closed circle nothing can pass; therefore problems should be solved in the daytime, during the period of the sun. The time before going to sleep is best to bring vibrations to a very high level through prayer or relaxing so deeply that the soul level is reached, but not to evaluate a difficult situation. If there is some decision to be made, tell your subconscious to work on it while your conscious mind is asleep. The subconscious never sleeps. Its safety valve is dreaming, without dreams we would all be mad, but besides dreaming there is plenty of time left for solving problems and it is good to give the subconscious work to do.

A team of doctors have at last penetrated part of the mystery surrounding sleep. Everyone's dreams are seen in a rapid eye movement, known as REM. Student volunteers, who offered themselves as guinea pigs, helped greatly in the findings of what dreams are all about.

They were divided into three groups, all of them attended a film consisting of cuttings about the German concentration camps at the end of the war and happenings in Japanese and Korean prisoner-of-war camps. The film showed man in his most cruel and sadistic state and no normal person could look at it without feeling sick and ashamed. The students were horrified and terribly upset as their generation knew very little about the abominations of war camps, they were totally unprepared, not knowing beforehand what the film was about.

After the film the first group was allowed to sleep the whole night. The second group was awakened each time they showed REM and the third group was kept awake the whole night. The next day, the same film was shown again, groups two and three reacted exactly the same as before; but the first group who had had a complete night's sleep, showed less anxiety and disturbance. This experiment was repeated many times with different groups and the results were always the same. The students who had slept undisturbed, adjusted, and rationalised the film.

This is exactly what happens to all our experiences in life. The average person digests in dreams the experiences of the day. In the dreams it is reasoned out and classified into the appropriate section of the subconscious; the ability or disability to do this is the difference between a reasonably balanced or an emotionally disturbed person.

Science is now trying to find a way to bring this adjustment about through inducing normal dream reaction in the mentally disturbed. Taking sleeping pills interferes to a large extent with the normal procedure. Drugs are confusing to the subconscious to such an extent, that it can no longer distinguish between fantasy and reality; and is therefore not able to do the work.

Man's nervous system has become more refined, especially in the last 2,000 years, as it goes parallel with the development of the intellect and soul. The vibrations of modern man cannot mix, unpunished, with the completely different and low vibrations of drugs. Hard drugs can completely shatter the nervous system, that is the etheric body, and not only damage it irreparably for the rest of this life, if the person survives the shock, but has an extensive influence on future incarnations.

> When Moreland first came to see me he had the vagueness and airiness of a hallucinatory drug-taker. He also dabbled, but to what extent I do not know, in black magic. He went on and off drugs and I never quite knew in what condition he would appear in class; I realised he needed round the clock contact, which I was unable to give him. I introduced him to a member of an esoteric, cultural society, who was willing to give him all the time he needed. Moreland is now one of the most active members of that society and is back at university.

The subconscious should be directed by the conscious mind, together they are an ideal team, they supplement each other to perfection. The human being has to use this combination consciously and if he does there is nothing beyond the reach of man in this world, not even is the sky the limit.

Only the Absolute is infallible. Even the most highly evolved person can make mistakes, but that does not invalidate the rest. It is up to each reader to think and ponder and assimilate what is acceptable to him. Even pure truth has to make sense to the intellect of the reader in order to be eventually integrated into his spirit-mind. Only what the latter accepts fully is then added for ever to the sum total of the knowledge — wisdom — soul of that being until the end of this evolution.

In exceptional cases a person can raise vibrations to the highest level. This is rather rare and can occur in certain circumstances, such as in a state of very deep meditation, through an act of faith and again in lifting the whole being above the occurring situation in a moment of great physical or mental suffering, pouring this whole emotion into love for God or mankind.

Shortly after World War Two, Anne, a continental woman, was unable to continue her trip to North-East India, as floods had covered the entire area. She reached a little village which was slightly above water level. From the first day it was obvious that something was very wrong, many people were so sick they could not move. Anne realised with horror that she was stranded in the middle of a cholera epidemic. The most sensible person in the village was an old Brahmin Priest, they both knew a smattering of Hindi, so they were able to communicate.

After the first moment of shock and with the help of the old Brahmin, Anne organised the village. She had all the patients brought to the biggest house to be nursed by the Brahmin and herself. The children were placed farthest away from the improvised hospital, with a handful of women to look after them and the Brahmin put the most trustworthy person in charge. The rest of the inhabitants were placed in another part of the village, with the village elders in charge. A group was to provide the food for everyone and another group brought new cases to the border of the compound and burned all the possessions of the sick.

Anyone who has seen cholera patients will understand the stress Anne went through, she was very fastidious and normally carried some boiled water with her, but this had now run out. She did not drink and ate only water-melon. She also had a repulsion against dirt, ugliness and disease and had been able to avoid these most of her life. Now as she saw all this tremendous and overwhelming suffering, something happened to her; she forgot her own self completely and had only one desire — to help. She devoted herself entirely to nursing. As death took its toll she did not want anyone to touch the dead, who were burnt in the traditional Indian manner, by the Brahmin and herself, on the side of the water.

One night going from patient to patient, her compassion rose to such heights that there and then she felt compelled to kneel down and pray. She was not in the habit of praying, having given it up in her teens, but on this hot and humid night with the foul, putrid smell all around, she experienced God. Everything around her disappeared and there was a bright, dazzling white light and in this light everything was connected with everything else, everyone linked with the other, united into oneness. All separateness had disappeared and everything had taken on the same value, the same importance. She did not know how long this experience lasted, but it seemed eternal. When it faded all tiredness had left her and she understood suffering. She also understood the wheel of life; to be born, to love, to suffer, to die was all part of it and the revolt against seemingly useless suffering had fallen away from her. Now that she knew and understood the work became much easier.

A few days later when a doctor and two nurses arrived from the U.N.O. she left without talking to them as the experience was still too vivid. The impression was lasting; she studied Yoga and devoted her time to teaching others.

In this New Age, mankind has to take a step forward in evolution and overcome that egotistic, self-centred, predatory state. Basically we are still like animals defending, to the death if necessary, every bit of property we have. There is no difference between a lion marking the boundaries of his territory by urinating, or a man building a fence around his property. Our wars are a typical example, the world has still to wake up to the fact that we do not own anything, what we have is rather lent to us by God and is meant to be shared. The world belongs equally to all its inhabitants. Everyone has the right to have a decent place in the sun. This goes not only for man, but also for animals and plants. The majority of people consider this a utopian idea, but their so-called realistic way has only brought disaster, wars, famine, disease, overpopulation and pollution. It is time to approach the problem from a new angle, to use the power of the mind linked with compassion.

One of the things the individual needs most today is the courage of his convictions. Basically most people are good, and would rather have a happy world around them. They like to help, but are very luke-warm about it. They do not make any special effort to help, they do not like to be noticed, they want to be like their neighbours, in fact the only thing they lack is the courage to be different, to acclaim openly that they want peace and internationality, that they want everyone to have a decent life. When at last they admit to themselves that they are old and have not lived up to their ideals, it is mostly too late in life.

The average person uses that wonderful power, the mind, very rarely. He may not agree because he considers that he thinks too much; he may think so much that he cannot even go to sleep at night. That is correct, except that what he calls thinking is not thinking at all; it is just compulsory association. The mind jumps, uncontrolled, from one thing to another, rarely dwelling on one thought for more than a fraction of a second. This makes it unproductive and more importantly, these so-called thoughts are not only useless, but worse, negative and destructive.

There is no point in going over the past in any form, as it has gone forever. A lot of people have the unfortunate habit of brooding over the past, about bygone things. An unpleasant remark from a family member or co-worker is not worth thinking about. It was probably made on the spur of the moment, unpremeditated, just an emotional reaction to something you had said earlier. It hurts only you because you take yourself much too seriously. Nothing can hurt us, unless we allow it to do so, we are completely free in our reactions, no one can force us to be upset, if we do not want to be.

Let us analyse this reaction we have to an unkind remark. What was said to us is either true or not true; most probably it is true, but exaggerated. In the latter case the observer does us a service by pointing out one of our shortcomings. Is it not said 'we learn by the enemy, not by the friends'? This gives us a chance to eliminate that fault. On the other hand, if it is not true, then why worry about it? A lot of people have wrong ideas about us, this is one more — what does it matter? We tend to take everything too personally, too egotistically.

Have you ever thought what the difference between unhappiness and happiness is? It has nothing whatsoever to do with material possessions, otherwise all rich people would be happy and the poor unhappy. It is rather the other way around. There are more happy poor people than rich ones. Why? Because happiness is a state of mind, a disposition, a state of being able to see things from a positive angle, and to accept circumstances, to enjoy life, to think pleasant thoughts — most of the time.

> I was having afternoon tea with my friend Nanette in her lovely garden. It was one of those peaceful summer days when time seems to stand still. My friend was unusually quiet and through the fragrance of Jasmin, I slipped into the past and I found myself in India. Martin, Nanette's youngest son brought me back to this world as he came running, laughing, and shouting towards us, followed by his yapping new puppy. He dropped on the lawn in front of us and with the puppy in his arms looked the picture of happiness. Then his expression became quiet and he said, as much to himself as to us, touching his chest lightly with his right hand, 'It is in here, it's all mine and no one can take it away from me'; and he continued to play with his little dog. We were both rather amazed that such a small child fully understood the meaning of happiness.

Very critical people have difficulty in being happy, because they are dissatisfied most of the time, trivial though the cause of their unhappiness may be. To be happy does not have to mean acceptance of each and every event. One can always change circumstances if one does not waste precious energy in lamentation, but use this energy for change to bring about the right conditions.

Nearly everyone has a kind of pet antagonist; wife, husband, children, in-laws, fellow workers and so on. To think of people when they are not present is, most of the time, useless and frustrating. At the first impact this may seem a rash, unfriendly statement, but if you check your thoughts over a few days you will be surprised how very rarely you think pure, loving thoughts. There is mostly some disapproval or at least a slight criticism.

Another negative use of the wonderful mind is day-dreaming. It is a very unhealthy form of escapism. Day-dreamers make up orgies of generosities and revenge, but all the time they are the heroes, faultless, the best beings of their kind on earth. This hero-worshipping of the self is so destructive, because it is so far removed from reality, from truth. It keeps the dreamer from changing his life for the better, as there is not enough energy left for real life.

The human being is at his best when realising his short-comings and then going ahead and improving himself. The deepest satisfaction comes from helping others, it does not matter in what way. There are practically as many ways as there are human beings because each person requires an individual approach.

The more one overcomes that self-centred, egotistical outlook on life, the less frustrating life becomes. A human life is evaluated by its help to others. Helping can be done in count-less ways, but one of the most beneficial is a happy, radiant personality, not just when it appears convenient, but all the time. Simple examples are:

To be friendly and relaxed in the waiting room of the dentist, when one is already late for work and there are still quite a few people ahead.
Not to be disturbed when wrongly accused of something we did not do, and not to defend ourselves because the important thing is that we know we did not do what we have been blamed for.
Not to be affected by the mannerism of a person in our surrounding and countless things which usually get on our nerves, if we let them.

On the sixth day of creation, God made man in his own image and endowed him with a special gift; to be master of this world, and to rule in God's name. To govern the world, man has first to learn to master himself, to use and apply the Great Forces of the Universe within himself. What are these Great Forces? Mind is mind-substance or that which is underlying the principle of the mind. Mind-substance was the first manifestation in Evolution. The western world considers mind as something vague with a rather metaphysical meaning, a condition rather than a thing. Not so in the philosophy of Yoga. In Yoga it is rather considered as a substance or essence, universal mind, all pervading, but not the Absolute, only the first of His emanations.

To know oneself is to be able to instantaneously recognise an idea-emotion as belonging to one of a group of four:

> For the good of mankind.
> Egotistic, hence indifferent or bad for mankind.
> Belonging to a world of fantasy.
> Belonging to the realm of memory — the past.

The instant correct classification of an idea is the mark of a very mature mind. Every idea is automatically identified as being pleasant or unpleasant, which is purely instinctive, a kind of projection of the ego. Worthwhile ideas should be executed immediately, or written down for later use. If we allow ideas to pass us by without using them, they get into the habit of evaporating, to be used by another being in deep concentration on a similar subject, as a hunch or brainwave. Similarly we often flinch from making an effort, and before we know it, the effort making quality is gone. The more we use our ideas, the more ideas stream in, and the less we use ideas, the less ideas we get.

We have to make an effort all the time, in being conscious of our wonderful ability and by preventing our minds from becoming vague and wandering. Every day we should make a few gratuitous efforts by way of self-discipline, even if they have no other meaning in themselves than discipline. A man is only free to the degree of his discipline.

We are transmitting all the time and are also on the receiving end continuously and we receive only on the wave-length to which we are tuned. This is the pattern in every way of life. For instance, on delivering a lecture, more important than the intellectual meaning of the words, or the literary style, are the circumstances under which it is transmitted and the spirituality and conviction of the speaker.

The conviction of the lecturer charges his words with such a strong vibration, that very few people in the audience will not respond. In reading, especially if you are very interested in the subject and therefore tuned in, your vibration will be as strong as your interest. The stronger your vibration, the deeper will be your understanding and absorption. Learning is best and quickest when we are emotionally involved. A child who loves his teacher learns far better and more easily than if this is not the case and if there is any animosity between teacher and pupil, there is very little absorption because of the emotional block. A sensitive child may be so disturbed by this situation that it will show in his physical condition. Some parents tend to get jealous of the teacher's influence on their child and they will stop short of nothing to undermine this relationship. If only they knew how they harm the child with this unnecessary interference.

The fixation of the human mind on a subject, whether it be positive or negative, concentrates it, and brings all the previous knowledge and memory to the surface, from the subconscious to consciousness. This applies to meditation, study, concentration, being tense and frustrated, absorbed in negative thoughts, worry and so on.

Through the rotation of a dynamo, electricity is produced. The same phenomenon happens through the concentration of the human mind on a particular subject. This 'rotation' produces vibrations of varying intensity, the highest being self-realisation. The consciousness of higher dimensions or enlightenment is only possible through that state of concentration and singlemindedness.

All discoveries are made through the force of concentration. All forces are vibratory, there is every range from the lowest to the highest. A higher vibration either neutralises or rejects a lower one when it is in opposition. If the lower vibration is much stronger it will gain the upper hand. Vibrations form waves in the atmospheric ether, some can be analysed, being in the analysable part of the atmosphere, others cannot. The strength, force, length and rapidity depend on the emotional force with which they are initially launched. As man is the highest being on this planet, he is able to produce a higher vibration than any other being.

When Joel recovered from the shock of the car accident, his first thought was his wife. He called her, there was no answer and looking around in the darkness he found her half buried underneath the upside-down car. Her eyes were closed and kneeling at her side a terrible feeling of guilt nearly suffocated him. An overwhelming desire to help her swept through him and in answer to his plea he felt an incredible strength. He sprung up and lifting the heavy car threw it over. Emma was badly hurt but after extensive surgery recovered completely. It is still a wonder to Joel how he could single-handedly do the job of four men.

Man is matter and as matter in itself has no weight, by the overcoming of gravity man will be able to walk on water, or float through air, as do all the planets, suns and stars. Without the magnetic pull there is no weight and the magnetic pull is limited to the sphere or the body itself. Once man can raise his vibrations above the earth's magnetic force, he can nullify its effects.

This knowledge was used by the sons of God, it was as natural to them as walking is to us. But now man has to acquire this knowledge through mastering the planetary forces. This will enable him to regain his birthright to become as in the image of God, to be perfect and eventually to merge with his source from whence he came.

There were giants in the earth in these days; and also after that, when the sons of God came in unto the daughters of men, and they bare children to them, the same became mighty men which were of old, men of renown.

Genesis Ch. 6: v. 4.

Concentration and Meditation

Before I start on the subject itself, I want to go into the very basis for all the mental disciplines.

The human being consists of the seven principles — the seven planes. We must differentiate between the three physical levels, which are the physcial body, the etheric body and the astral body, and the four mental levels, which consist of the instinctive mind or subconscious, the intellect or conscious mind, the superconscious mind or soul which is also known as intuition and at the very top of this scale we find pure SPIRIT.

Each separate being contains all seven planes of the Universe, in a latent form, from the beginning.

Let us examine the three physical levels. Of them all, the characteristics of the physical body are best known to us and need not be discussed in detail. Hatha Yoga, physical culture and sports, deal largely with the maintenance and tuning up of our body, in order that we may use it to its fullest extent. The physical body is such a wonderful piece of machinery, that we cannot help but marvel at the precision and intricacy of its mechanism. We should always enjoy looking after it.

In this physical world, on this physical planet which is condensed to the most concentrated point of manifested matter, we have to have a physical vehicle in order to gather experiences. Its very density and limitation within three dimensions set the requirements for contact with a maximum amount of friction. Friction is necessary for advancement; without resistance of some kind there is no need for an expenditure of effort.

The subject of the etheric, pranic body is a most stupendous and far-reaching one. (See chapter on etheric body.)

However, since we want to get on to the subject of concentration and meditation, it is sufficient, at this stage, to mention that a good understanding of prana and breathing technique is a pre-requisite to all mental disciplines. No person who has learned anything about prana need ever be lacking in it. After all, this is life-force, this vital substance, is everywhere, in everything, all-pervading.

Prana is in the air all around us, a sparkling, mysterious force which permeates every atom and is the basis of its atomic life. Out of the universal storehouse of prana — energy — life-force, everyone may draw as much as they need. The technique for doing so, is very simple, the reservoir is always full, what a wealth of strength and energy we have at our disposal.

The astral body is a replica of our physical shape, constructed of very much finer matter and therefore not restricted by the limitations of space and time. In actual size it is slightly bigger. It is the part of us which separates independently during sleep and may be seen to hover over a person at the time of death.

Let us now look at the lowest of the mental principles — the instinctive mind: We share the instinctive mind with the animal kingdom where, in its most basic form, it constitutes the instinct of survival. In fact, instinct is the key from the third, the animal kingdom, to the fourth, the human kingdom, just as the intellect or mind is the key from the fourth into the fifth or spiritual kingdom.

On each level a form of individualisation takes place. The instinctive mind governs our reaction to light and dark; heat and cold; pain, hunger, thirst, and all the friction of daily life. As a form of survival, it developed the fighting instinct, aggression as well as defence, and the nesting instinct. Both are still very strong in man, and we know many examples of super-nest building and protective aggressiveness in our friends, even if we have more difficulty in detecting them in ourselves.

We delegate a lot of everyday tasks to our instinctive mind, and by creating habit patterns, which can be governed entirely by instinct, we leave our intellect free for more important tasks. In fact if we disturb these habit patterns, by interference of thinking, we quite often make mistakes. For instance, driving a car; when you try to teach someone to drive, you concentrate on, and explain, each separate movement and pedal and you will most likely end up grating the gears or forgetting something simple which is normally done automatically.

Concentration is an exercise and discipline of the intellect or conscious mind. In concentration we learn to isolate the thinking process at a particular time, we learn to discipline ourselves to think of nothing apart from the subject of concentration. We become aware of our intellect as a brilliant instrument which we are privileged to use, in connection with free will, because it is our free will which chooses the subject of concentration. Once we are able to stop thinking at will, at any time we like, we have made one of the most important steps forward. Not only can we then interrupt wrongful thinking, criticism or worrying, but we can instantaneously switch to the right thought.

Intellect is the middle level between instinct and intuition. It is ours to use as we like, and the result of our use or misuse of it is called Karma. The law of Karma, the law of cause and effect, works according to whether we use our intellect to underline our instincts and further our purely personal, egocentric ambitions, or whether we use the intellect to make contact with our super mind and so further our evolution. At first this may seem to be a purely personal, egocentric ambition — until we remember that we are all part of one enormous whole and that the evolving of even a single unit must necessarily effect the evolution of the whole.

Animals do not possess intellect. Intellect is an aspect of individualisation and marks the transition from the group souls of the lower third kingdom to the single soul in the fourth higher one. Intellect is vital for advancement up to a very high level of evolution when it is eventually integrated into the super mind of a very advanced individual.

The intuitional level has absorbed the very essence of gathered knowledge, stripped of emotions and egotistic tendencies. Knowledge has been distilled and refined to become wisdom. The store of wisdom is permanent, carried over from life to life, an attribute of our Soul in its quest for evolution.

We know comparatively little about the super mind, except that it is the vehicle for our soul and the seat of our Individuality as compared to our Personality which is tied up with the instinctive mind and intellect. Let us remember that personality is temporary and coloured by the limitations of our instincts. Individuality on the other hand is indestructible and stays with us during an evolutionary cycle. It is added to each life and forms the basis for the level of the next life, by supplying us, at the very outset, with traits, talents and characteristics in our unfolding personality.

There is a good reason why we do not remember everything that has been learned and stored in other lives. Such a memory would interfere with the decisions and attitudes we take to given circumstances and tests. It would interfere with our free will.

> The highest mental principle, Spirit, is far beyond our comprehension. Let us just remember here, that Spirit is the divine spark within each one of us, a tiny fragment of the Universal Spirit. It is non-dual, without attributes, neither positive or negative, male or female, good or bad. Spirit is unmanifest and for that reason, beyond description or comprehension. It is that tiny part of us which makes us members of a Universal Brotherhood of all living things. It is that part which qualifies us for the title, 'Gods in the making'.

Let us now look at the discipline of Concentration. We have already established the fact that it is entirely a function of the Intellect or Conscious Mind. It is an active form of mental exercise, being able to focus on one particular, concrete subject at first, and later on an abstract idea.

By concentrating on a subject, we make ourselves aware of every detail of that subject. We note the size and shape and texture — we use our memory to dig up details of its origin and relative values. By focusing our whole attention on one line of thought, we open a valve in our minds, a very selective valve similar to the tuner on a television or radio receiver. Suddenly a great rush of all the relevant information comes tumbling into our consciousness. We are astonished at our intimate knowledge, we marvel at the detail which our senses have picked up without our registering it, and which they have passed on to our memory. What started as a duty and exercise performed as a pre-requisite for meditation, has turned into a satisfying and revealing experience.

With all these facts fresh in the mind, do a short concentration exercise.

To start with, it is necessary to have as much bodily comfort as possible. If your body is comfortable, its aches and twinges will not distract the attention. What we want to achieve is the basic comfort of a straight back, relaxed shoulders, where each vertebrae is supporting the one above it and is itself resting squarely on the one below. Where there is no tension in the neck and the breathing becomes slow, and effortless. In fact, a perfect posture, which is so right we cannot help smiling.

Start with a breathing exercise which lengthens the breath and establishes a state of peace. Inhale to a count of four and exhale to a count of eight. Check that your shoulders are really relaxed and that there is no frown between the eyebrows. Establish the rhythm of your breath: IN — four pulse beats: OUT — eight pulse beats. Keep your mind occupied with the gentle ebb and flow of your breath. Be aware of the fact that you do not only TAKE IN breath, prana, life-force, but that you GIVE OUT in double measure.

When you are fully absorbed by the rhythm of breathing you can shift your mind to concentrate on yesterday's action. Recollect your motives and view them from a universal standpoint.

Repeat this procedure till you feel the influence of your concentration in your more thoughtful actions. When you become aware of conscious living it is time to go a step further and start with short meditation.

There is, for many people, a very narrow division between concentration and meditation, and during certain concentration exercises it is quite possible to slip into meditation.

To define the difference — in meditation we open the tuner in our mind once again — but this time it is directed towards our Super Mind or Soul. We become recipients of thought patterns, mostly those which we have formed ourselves over long periods.

For meditation we need absolute physical and mental stillness. We must learn to become passive, still and humble. This must, however, not be confused with just 'sitting and thinking'; there is nothing lazy about meditation. Initially it requires enormous discipline and concentration in order to find contact with our intuition.

As long as random thoughts appear within our consciousness, as long as we are bound by subconscious or conscious stimuli, there is no chance of meditation. Both Instinctive Mind and Intellect must be mastered and put to rest and this might take months, depending on the strength of our will.

The question will no doubt arise, that if meditation is such a difficult thing to achieve in our present state of evolution, why not be content with learning to concentrate, as this also allows us an entrance into the great library of our accumulated knowledge and experience? Do we really need to achieve meditation? This question must be solved individually after having been successful with relaxation. You may be happy and satisfied and leave it at that, or you may want to probe deeper.

Because the effort of each single unit towards advancement in evolution does, and must, effect the level of evolution on the whole, we can, by living consciously and devoting our lives to helping mankind establish through the exercise of our own free will another bridge between personality and individuality.

Meditation is the means to become what you want to be. It is communication with God — from God towards Man, while prayer is, the other way round, communicating from Man towards God.

In meditation the Higher Consciousness is contacted. By quieting the physical body and the emotions the Innermost is reached. It is going inwards from the outside — working from the periphery to the centre. From the intellectual mind to the Spirit Mind, from the objective mind to the subjective mind. This is the reason for our being born on Earth; we need the physical body as vehicle for the work.

To achieve the best results in meditation one must be able to hold one-pointed concentration. In addition to this, infinite patience is required. Meditation must become a daily habit, a training to leave all preoccupations behind, to create such an inner stillness that the deeper region in us can open up and little by little allow the superconsciousness to express itself. This is what yoga teaches us to do. Meditation is a wonderful gift bestowed on mankind. Through it we slowly learn to understand the hidden sense of our life, the purpose behind the seemingly meaningless happenings of our days and we learn liberation from the countless external needs.

Meditation is the most successful if you are motivated by a burning desire to reach union with the Absolute. If it is coupled by regularity and stillness you will infallibly reach your aim — God-realisation.

As you will recall from the chapter on relaxation, it is important to start as early as possible in life to relax progressively and to get consciousness to rise from the subconscious to the conscious level. No matter what happens to a person who is in the habit of relaxing or meditating, there will never be that feeling of futility, of being lost, because with a degree of proficiency the flow of consciousness can be directed wherever desired. For example: after having devoted her entire life to looking after her family a mother feels absolutely lost when she is left alone through circumstances involving the marriage of her children, the death of her husband and so on. Why? She neglected her own soul. Never having adopted the habit of going within herself, all her actions were external, the flow of her whole life was external, so if every facet of that external flow is gone there is only emptiness left behind. But, if the person has the habit of turning inwards daily, the flow of life is eternal and can be directed into other channels. The choice of the new direction to be adopted lies entirely with the person and this can be done over and over again; the internal growth and development is never interrupted.

The best results in meditation are achieved after having mastered unwavering one-mindedness for at least ten minutes. It is essential not to be disturbed; it is also very helpful to always select the same place, one, where for preference, there is no distraction, where there are objects which have nothing to do with the necessities of daily life and the speed of present day living, a kind of sanctuary as it were.

Meditation is one of the vital methods prescribed by Raja Yoga to develop your mind power, and thereby raise the degree of spirituality. The best way is to sit cross-legged in the full or half lotus position but this is not essential. If you are not used to sitting this way for any length of time, choose a hard chair, low enough for your feet to rest easily on the floor. Keep a very erect spine. Make no violent effort to control the mind, but rather allow it to exhaust itself by gradually unwinding. It will run wild first, taking every advantage of

the opportunity. But after a few weeks, the time of running
wild will be shorter each time.

When the mind is quiet and calm, fix your attention on the
'I - AM', using these two words as a mantram, this being just
one of innumerable meditative practices.

Mantrams are the sounds of the heart. It can be heard by
the ear, but it does not necessarily have to have a meaning for
the mind. Mantram is the power of the sacred speech in
which the transcendental sound of the Spirit that dwells in
the human heart is perceived, intuitively, in the Super Mind.
Mantrams are connected with the vibration of the elements;
together with prayers, but independent of each other, they are
invoking the blessings of God and the beneficial forces of the
universe present in the elements of air, fire, water and earth.
The elements support our life and serve us in the accomplishment of our work. We can use Mantrams in daily life during
our routine work; by doing so we saturate everything in us
and around us with the Mantram, with the idea of the Mantram.

After you have learned to quieten the mind to some degree
you will become conscious of your inner world. Some see, in
the beginning, flickering lights or they realise that in spite
of being still there are muffled thoughts. These will eventually
cease and it is not unusual to then see coloured, or black and
white pictures. They come from the subconscious which in a
way is like talking; the subconscious is not willing to give in
lightly. This is not important though, and one should not
waste time worrying over it; nevertheless try to rise above
the pictures. A good way is to imagine to rise to the crown
of the head. Eventually you will see a very bright dazzling
white light. Sit as long as you can, just being in that light.
This is the beginning of union with your soul and clears the
subconscious of fear.

> It is often possible, but not necessary, to see a bright
> light between the eyebrows. That light is surrounded by
> a blue inner circle and a golden outer one. This is the
> Trinity.
> The inner-most brilliant light — the God-father-principle;
> the blue light — the Holy-spirit-mother-principle;
> and the golden outer ring — the Son-principle.

This is an expansion of consciousness and comes after some
testing of your faith. One never knows in advance such a

testing. Sometimes it is not even realised that such a test has been passed. During this expansion of consciousness try to merge with the golden light till you can hear the steady roar of creation (Shabda-Logos — the word). Then go into the blue light and you will expand into the universal understanding of the Mother-principle and last break through into the pure white light, to become part of it and to understand the source of all being and of the universe.

Each time you can achieve this your consciousness expands permanently a little further. The more often you succeed the greater will become your understanding of the world in addition to fostering the development of your inner powers, and your own special psychic gifts. The more steady and regular your meditation, the better the results.

When the highest stage of meditation is reached there is no longer a need for a special position, time or ritual because a condition of constant meditation is reached and the perfect state of total living in the present is achieved.

Every act is guided from within through inspiration. This living in the present and being the channel of God's plan can only be achieved through unconditional surrender of the Personality to God — the Absolute. All personal desire has to be overcome in order to succeed in an uninterrupted contact with the universal mind.

Breathing with mantram: very beneficial for meditation, — a source of continuous strength.

Om is the symbol for the Absolute — the Infinite-sunyata of the Buddhist — and is only used in meditation.

Om Mani Padme Hum is pronounced: Om manee peme houm.

There is a special way to use this mantram:

O is short	two seconds.
M is longest	twelve seconds.
Ma is short	two seconds.
Nee is short	two seconds.
Pe is short	two seconds.
Me is short	two seconds.
Houm is long	six seconds.

Inhale and as you exhale as slowly as you can, chant on low notes the mantram. Use the Tibetan mala (rosary) for counting and breath.　　Start with seven breaths and with the time do as many as you like.

Om mani padme hum means approximately — the jewel in the heart, the Christ in the heart, He who is the perfect image of what we will be in the faraway future.

Om	Wisdom of universal law.
Mani	Wisdom of equality (the jewel)
Padme	Wisdom of discrimination and vision
Hum	Great mirror of the self.

Om	= The Absolute		
Mani	= Akasha	=	Tamas
Padme	= Lotus	=	Rajas
Hum	= The sacrifice of self	=	Sattwa

Hamsa (Ahamsa)	I am He
Sa ham	He (is) I
Hamsa	Inhale: Ham, exhale: Sa.

Exhale double the amount of the inhalation.

Sa ham	Inhale come with your mind up the spine from the solar plexus to the throat, exhale go with your mind down the spine. Repeat till you have a steady rhythm then you do not think of the breath any more.　Your whole attention is in the spine going up and down with the consciousness.
Om Satyam	God is truth Be with your mind in the heart and repeat the mantram without consideration of breath.
Aham Brahmasmi	I am God Concentrate in the head, recite the mantram without pause. Breathe normally.

If Om is used silently, inhale think O, exhale think M.　You can place the Om in the heart or in the head centre.

For chanting the Om inhale silently and exhale sounding the Om, first half O, second half M. . .　　. . like this:

OOOOOOOOOOOOOOOOOOMMMMMMMM MMMMMMMMM

Fragments from Students'
Meditation Experiences

M.S., convinced of the value of the new technique of transcendental meditation taught by the Yogi Maharishi Mahesh, advised me to take advantage of his visit and be initiated. I liked the idea of a direct, deep-thrust technique to match our modern, fast age.

But two things repelled me, one, his rather dogmatic assertion that this system is the only one that should be taught, and his voice which became rather high-pitched towards the end of the lecture in the Town Hall. I was very dubious whether to go ahead or not.

On the night of the initiation, the moment I entered where he sat cross-legged on a couch, I felt a wonderful calm in the room, his voice was vibrant and low. Peace and well-being emanated from his presence. I understood then something M.S. had told us about her own master in India. She had said it was a marvellous feeling just to be near him. I had wondered what could be so marvellous about being near an old, old man on a lonely mountain? Maharishi Mahesh is a comparatively young man yet, but the atmosphere he radiated affected one powerfully.

Have since mentally repeated the sound given in initiation twice daily during meditation. The mental repetition of the word is to lead thought deeper and deeper till the word or sound disappears and it has reached its source or, as he calls it, the Absolute. Then one carries back into one's daily activities the power gained from this 'dive'.

The success of one's 'diving' is to be gauged by the smooth success of one's work and daily life or otherwise.

To know what goes on when going to a deeper level, the

mind must be developed to a fine sharpness and this is brought about by practice.

During one meditation I lost the word, became unaware, thus showing my mind is not fine enough yet, but then with my inner ear heard a complete story suitable for children of kindergarten age. I typed it out immediately afterwards.

Today near the end of meditation, the sound was not a sound so much as flickers or sparks.

When starting to sound the word mentally felt the impulse of the tongue to go into position to form the word and, though the tongue did not actually move, the attention focused there.

Felt tense afterwards so tried to recollect where I had gone wrong: I had observed the word with close attention, thus putting myself on one side and the word on the other. Exactly the wrong thing and the opposite of what we had been told, to let the word come and to let it go easily. He had stressed this point so many times, that it should be effortless, without straining, that it is a wonder I forgot.

Thoughts while meditating on the sound lum: Love, Liebe: L'amour actually contains the sound. Is it the sound for reproduction of human beings only, or all things on earth? I rather think yes, it is for all new creation. Orgasm, an instant of deepened sharing of life force and if conception takes place it enables the seed of the new form to live. It gives life to the new concept.

After the auto-suggestion of cold and then warm: I had a feeling of expansion and the feeling of something limitless breathing me. I was like an onlooker, there was one part of me looking and the other part being breathed by something greater than I could understand. The air was flowing through me in a way, as if I was not there, or as if I was made from some type of porous material, and the flow was from the feet to the head; all the pores were open, especially in the face, feet and hands. The air was very invigorating and just lying there I felt every cell of my body tingling with an extra unknown quality. My body felt floatingly light and wonderfully flexible and that if I was to do anything it would be perfect; I just knew this.

Then I felt my mind expanding, it was not visible, but very real and the expansion continued till I was conscious of the whole Universe; what a delight, what a bliss. I was not a person, I was the whole Universe. I do not know how long this state lasted. But after a while I felt my body and I realised I was a person again. Very reluctantly I got up as I had work to do.

When I sat at my writing desk my ideas just streamed out into my pen and in no time I had written an article which needed no correction and was considered one of my best.

G.D.

> Like the Swan
> gliding serenely over the water
> I have believed
> My own reflection
> In the unbroken surface ahead.
>
> Like the Swan
> I work and move frantically
> Below the surface —
> But the result of such action
> Shows only where I have passed.

B.M.

After three weeks of very consistent meditation and the repetition of 'Om mani padme hum' I had a vivid and unforgettable experience during relaxation. My awareness was only in the eyebrow centre and I could 'look' along my outstretched body which seemed to go on and on towards my toes in the manner of a surrealist painting. I heard a male voice first from a space next to my right ear which was drawn in space like an eastern brush painting with bold, free strokes. Then I heard the same deep voice from a triangle which was suspended next to my left ear. I could not make out the words and when I became too eager to understand, both shapes vanished. Only a slightly curved, earth textured line stayed for a while across my chest.

In this relaxation I saw a solid, striped shape, rather like a wooden gym-horse which was shaded from yellow at the wide base, through gold, ochre, orange and olive green towards the flat narrow top. Behind it was another, larger triangular shape, translucent and vaguely mustard yellow striped. I realised that the smaller, solid shape was I, being led by the larger triangle like a child is led by the hand. It was a pleasant, secure feeling.

At first I felt the upper part of my body expanding until I was sure that I was touching something with my left shoulder and upper arm. (The person next to me was too far away to be in physical contact.) Then a brilliant light above my face, which felt warm like sunshine, grew until it was circled by the colours of the rainbow. Not hard-edged circles, but diffused — one into the other. The very edges were like a fringe. As soon as I registered this intellectually it disappeared although the feeling of expansion stayed on.

Before I started Yoga I had two very strong fears which I could not overcome by will-power alone and which left me after I had become sufficiently relaxed and positive not to project my morbid imagination into a basic dislike. I believe that it is part of our very human composition that we have sympathies and antipathies towards certain animals, movements, foods, climates, etc., we can either 'feed' these until they grow out of all proportion and into phobias or we can recognise them, accept them and make the best of them when the necessity arises.

I hated spiders ever since one of them fell through the wooden ceiling of an Austrian peasant house and onto my cot where it sat facing me on the slope of my feather bed and I was sure it would slide towards my face. I still have no desire to make a pet of a tarantula and those hairy legs and bulbous eyes on stalks are not my idea of beauty. But I can get within inches of one — if necessary — and be gentle about persuading it to leave my car or my room. I've come to terms with the fact that spiders are useful, that their constructions, including their book lungs and multiple stomachs are a marvel of nature.

I was petrified of flying and each trip was such a strain that I took some time to recover. I listened to every slightest variation in the noise of the engines, I imagined lightning bolts in every cloud, birds being sucked into the turbines, failures of every kind. Both take-off and landing were torture ever since a tyre burst on my very first flight just after the war. Being blessed with much imagination and an aeronautical husband who fed me technical data I concocted whole horror stories without realising it. What changed it? A kind of miracle just before a long overseas flight. The sudden realisation of my own vulnerability, of being a tiny part in a big scheme of things and having no right or reason to fear for myself when all around me were hundreds of other people with enough faith and trust to take such a trip.

I am free now, I love travelling and I am grateful for having been so afraid once because there are always people who still battle this same fear and who are quite happy to hold one's hand on take-off or landing or have someone smile at them when the tears of fright come into their eyes.

B.G.

With thanks to Margrit Segesman

In another world
Amongst the mists of Olympus
In another, similar world
You gave a promise . . .

Many lives passed
In many differing bodies
On many differing mountains
Your promise remained.

Dimly remembered
Veiled by permits of the senses
Glimpsed in times of great need
Your promise remained.

In a similar school
Once more dedicated to learning
You have answered my cry
As you promised.

Discharging your vows
Freeing us both from bondage
We now move on parallel paths
Towards a mutual goal.

B.M.

149

The Bioplastic Body and Findings of Russian Scientists

Since time immemorial the human race has been pondering about the nature of man and the source of his life. Many are the names given to this mysterious, all pervading universal force:

> The ancient Chinese called it — Vital Energy, Yin-Yang.
> The ancient Indians named it — Prana, Life-force, Akasha.
> Sir Isaac Newton used the word — Ether: the inter-related ocean of energy of this planet.
> The Russians of today give it the name — Bioplastic Body.
> The modern esotericist has adopted all of the above-mentioned terms:
> Akasha, Prana, Life-force, Vital Energy, Yin-Yang, Etheric Body and Bioplastic Body. There are many more expressions used today like: Energy-body, Beta-body, Counterpart-body, Pre-physical-body, etcetera.

Just after the Second World War I read about the Russian interest in ESP and their research on the human aura. From then on I collected available data from all countries concerned with scientific tests on ESP. By far the most daring and advanced in the field was the Soviet Union. From behind the Iron Curtain came exciting and startling news of work done on the Bioplastic Body, Cybernetic Psychology, Telepathy, Acupuncture and Psychic Healing.

There is no doubt about the veracity of this news. These reports also serve to confirm the well-known viewing of clairvoyants. Long before Christian saints and holy men were depicted with misty auras and golden halos around them, there already existed similar wall paintings from pre-historic times.

Very early in their studies of ESP the Soviet scientists deduced the Bioplastic Body. They tried for years, rather unsuccessfully, to photograph it. It took a complete outsider, S. D. Kirlian, an electrical engineer, to stumble quite by accident, upon a device to achieve the aim. This ingenious man, helped by his wife, Valentina, discovered a procedure to take pictures of the Bioplastic Body. He improved his own invention by more than a dozen patents and he still continues to improve upon it.

A high frequency spark oscillator that generates 75,000 to 200,000 electrical oscillations per second is connected with optical instruments, microscopes or electron-microscopes. There is no camera needed, as the object of research is placed between the oscillator and the photographic paper. The strong luminescence projects the picture of the Bioplastic Body on the paper.

The Bioplastic Body is a framework in the physical body. It is a scaffolding within the human body and fills every cell of it even surpassing the periphery of the skin and forming a radiant aura around it. Through this etheric framework the dense physical body is sustained. In case of sickness some of the channels get clogged, causing a faulty circulation.

Here are some of the incredible range of Russian findings becoming known to the Western world:
Every human being has his own individual Bioplastic Body which can always be recognised as such. Even if the physical appearance would be unrecognisable the aura would not change its basic individual pattern and could be recognised in any part of that organism, be it a finger of a man, a leaf of a tree or part of an animal.

The aura is also the most precise indicator of the slightest emotional disturbance. It shows sickness and deficiency of the metabolism long before any scientific test can trace it. This applies to every living organism.

Deep efficient breathing shows the picture of a healthy, luminous Bioplastic Body. The effect of a faulty breathing technique is a less vital aura. People who live in polluted areas have dimmer less radiant auras. The Bioplastic Body does not alter its individual basic pattern and sickness, fear, nervous disorder or any other change is super-imposed on the original auric structure.

In the photographing of telepathic reaction it is evident that the relaxed person is a good sender and receiver. The deep-feeling, serene individual rates by far the best.

Acupuncture works on the Bioplastic Body. It is used to bring back an even flow in the etheric network. The needles are inserted in the crosspoints of the web to activate the flow of life-force. Under the oscillator the Bioplastic Body indicates the points where the needles have to be placed.

The Soviet Union realised the far-fetching consequences of these extraordinary findings and already in the thirties set up funds for research on ESP. Last year the sum of twenty million dollars was used on the project and top scientists are working on it.

The Etheric Body

Ether and akasha are often taken as one and the same, but they are two different aspects of the same substance. Ether is a material quality compared with akasha which is a spiritual dimension — the mysterious fount of life to all beings. Akasha is the universal infinite mind containing all ideas, and ether is matter out of which all ideas are formed.

Akasha is the all-pervading ocean of every existing idea. Through inspiration man becomes conscious of a special idea. Desire to create is born and with the help of will a whirlpool starts in akasha, building an exact mould of the present idea and as ether flows into it the idea is cast. This applies in the physical as well as in the abstract world. Through this mental process the idea becomes so clear that it can be formulated — written or spoken, put to music, expressed in any possible art form or reproduced in any material form.

The form leaving akasha is like the act of birth — birth being the separation from the original source of gestation. Through the separation of the soul from the akashic substance comes consciousness. Consciousness brings about differentiation which, in turn, leads to individualisation of each separate body, be it an atom, a man, a star or a galaxy — as a child separates from the mother, establishing his own individuality and beginning his own personal life.

From the very beginning each individual being contains in latent form all seven planes of the Universe. Until the child is grown up he is linked in an intangible way with his mother. One after the other the separations occur, giving the growing child an opportunity to adjust to each new situation.

Birth	physical separation
Walking	etheric separation
School	mental separation
Puberty	emotional separation

In the next few years emotional maturity should take place. The demanding love of a child for his mother sublimated into an altruistic love for a friend, thus emotionally freeing him from her influence and thereafter he is ready for adult love with a contemporary partner of his own age group.

A premature severance of the natural relationship between mother and child results in a deep emotional insecurity. The younger the child, the more lasting the damage. The same happens in a slightly lesser degree, by the separation from the father or any parental substitute.

In our computerised time, the incredible advancement of science has destroyed in the vast majority of mankind, the capacity to stand in awe before the wonder of creation. People have lost the profound feeling of unity which comes from the understanding that everything existing uses the same life-force — that a little grub in the garden, as well as a highly evolved man, is part of the universal force and lives by it.

Ether is the bond between all living beings, macroscopic and microscopic. Man's etheric body consists of thousands and thousands of miles of pranic channels holding together the astral, mental and soul levels, shaping the physical body to an exact counterpart of the soul, surrounding it with a sort of protective bubble, thus separating it by a very fine boundary from the rest of the physical world.

The etheric body receives prana, or life-force, in this sequence: heart centre — solar plexus — etheric spleen. After having circulated three times through these centres, prana penetrates all the other centres and the whole etheric network, before being released into the physical body. It is then sent, enriched by the quality of the respective individual, into the universe. Ether is four-fold and each entity absorbs only the quality according to his evolutionary standard. Each man colours the released prana with his own spiritual level and by so doing adds positiveness or negativeness to the world.

There is a constant flow of force, from the highest to the lowest level, transmitting new and better ideas; all being impressed from above and passing on downwards after the great universal law of give and take.

This interaction goes on continuously from the solar logos — to our planet Earth — to man — to animal — to vegetable — to mineral. Every being is thus consciously or unconsciously involved in evolution and responsible for the state of affairs of our world.

The etheric body is extremely sensitive to emotion. It registers the slightest change in mood long before the conscious mind is aware of it. This sensitivity affects man both ways — positive or negative. Contentment, creativeness or any positive emotion accelerates the distribution of life-force, and health and well-being increase. On the other hand all strain and negative emotions influence, according to their strengths, the absorption of prana, thus endangering the person's health. The bloodstream immediately registers the lack of sufficient life-force, and exhaustion or sickness occur.

Apart from emotional disturbances the etheric body is also affected by living in an overpopulated or polluted area. Another cause of deficiency can be physical, i.e. emphysema, congestion of the respiratory tract or destruction of lung tissue through illness. There is a kind of static over-sensitiveness which prevents the etheric body from being well anchored in the physical body. This results in low vitality, very little resilience and a constant precarious state of health. It is the consequence of family upheavals in the first three years of a child.

In the union of man and woman, the purer the etheric body the greater the impact; the higher will the united souls rise, giving a very evolved soul the chance to incarnate. If sex is abused and made something very commonplace the flight of the united souls will not be able to reach as high.

A pure etheric body which works perfectly should be our aim. This involves certain definite requirements — the tuning in to higher vibrations and, by so doing, elimination of the lower levels. This is essential as it is impossible for those of coarser bodies to contact higher planes. It is not possible for the soul to use a coarse physical body for the transmission of spiritual knowledge. The loftier currents of thought cannot impress the little evolved brain. Hence, the refinement of the physical body is essential.

A daily session of hatha yoga, physical culture, or sport is a necessity, and should be done at the same time each day.

The use of plenty of water, both externally and internally is vitally required. Five to six hours sleep, with wide open windows, are enough as too much depletes the etheric body.

Another important point is correct diet. Careful judgment shown in the choice of food, wise refraining from heavy eating, and small amounts of good pure food perfectly assimilated are all that a human being requires. We should prefer:

> Unprocessed and unrefined food, such as pure honey, unpolished rice, raw sugar, crude olive oil, and stone ground flour; milk, yoghurt, whole wheat bread, all the vegetables grown above the ground that contain the sun, all fresh fruit, dried fruits and nuts, with the exception of peanuts because of their over-acidity. One of the greatest protections for the etheric body is the intake of natural vitamins. The ideal weight is that slightly less than the health charts stipulate; and, of course, you get a much better deal with a life assurance company if, apart from being fit, you are a little underweight.

Contact with the sun in working or walking, should be much sought after; and the vitalization that comes through its rays. The sun kills germs and frees us from disease. Sunbathing should not be done for more than half an hour on each side at a time.

When these requirements are attended to adequately, a definite process of elimination proceeds, and in the course of a few months the whole physical body shifts its polarisation gradually upwards, until, ultimately, you will have a body of higher vibrations.

The refining of the emotional body requires a different approach. The emotional body is simply a great reflector, it reflects the surroundings, it receives the impact of every passing desire. It contracts every whim and fancy in its environment. Every current sets it in motion and every sound causes vibrations, unless we are conscious of it and we inhibit this state of affairs and train ourselves to be selective, to register only the higher impressions. The goal of the advancing student should be to so train the emotional body that it will become as still and clear as a mirror, so that it may reflect perfectly and consciously only the higher mental level.

Most people are the playball of their own emotions, and even worse, the playball of the emotions of their surroundings; this is a state of personality level. To follow the desires of our higher self, and to be unruffled by the outside world should be our aim.

We should develop an awareness of those desires, motives and wishes that cross the emotional mind and select the ones of the higher level and inhibit the ones of the lower.

To facilitate this we should install definite periods of daily stilling of the emotional body in our everyday lives — taking all opportunities for stillness as they occur in our daily routine and even when going about our work. The destructive habit of continuously thinking ahead must be got rid of and replaced by concentration on the actual task at hand.

Meditate after stilling the mind with pranayamas. Through this you will overcome your sensitiveness to public opinion and vibration, and with time you will impose your own peaceful radiation on others.

Remember that the work is gradual and the steadier you are in your daily application, the greater the advancement. When you miss a day, you slide back several days; that is one of the reasons why some people do not advance, get tired and give up. It is better to have a short meditation daily, than an hour occasionally. If you meditate regularly any extension will be of benefit. For all improvement, steadiness and regularity are the cornerstone of your advancement.

To be successful in working on the mental body several things are essential:

> Clear thinking — not just on a subject you are especially interested in, but on all matters concerning man. To follow one thought to the exclusion of all other.
>
> The ability to still the mental body — so that thoughts from the highest abstract level, and from the intuitional level, can find a receptive sheet on which to impress themselves. This requires determined practice carried out regularly.
>
> Progress is made without undue self-analysis. As a wise man said: 'Pull not yourself up by the roots to see if there is growth'.

The seventy-seven centres in the etheric body:

The seven main centres are called: Chakras — Padmas — Lotuses — Wheels — Whirlpools.

Muladhara	at the base of the spine	Earth
Swadhisthana	halfway between the base of the spine and the navel	Water
Manipura	at the level of the kidneys	Fire
Anahata	at the level of the heart	Air
Vishuddhi	at the level of the throat	Ether
Ajna	at the level of the eyebrows	Akasha
Sahasrara	below the crown	Spirit

The twenty-one secondary centres:

In front of each ear, close to where the jawbones are connected.

Just above each of the two breasts.

Where the breastbones meet, close to the thyroid gland. (This with the two breast centres makes a triangle of force.)

In the centre of the palm of each hand.

In the centre of each footsole.

Just behind each eye.

On the level of the gonads. (The only ones to be on a different level in man and woman).

A little to the right on the level of the liver.

On the exit of the stomach.

Superimposed one on the other forming, therefore, one centre for the spleen.

On the back of each knee.

In the middle of the body, just a bit below the end of the chestbone. This, of all the twenty-one, is the strongest; and is closely related to the vagus nerve.

Close to the solar plexus, thus making a second triangle, this time below the diaphragm. (Sacral centre, solar plexus, base of the spine).

The forty-nine minor centres:

On the tip of each finger.

Between each of the fingers.

Two on the base of each hand.

On the tip of each toe.

Between each of the toes.

On either side of each ankle.

On each temple.

In the hollow of the base of the skull.

On each elbow.

The use of the centres as pressure points to cure is a science in itself. To give an understanding of the importance of the etheric body and its centres here are examples describing the use of two points:

To get rid of a headache or migraine use the centre in the hollow at the base of the skull. This can be done alone, but it is better to be helped by another person. Relax and look straight ahead with the chin down. The assistant stands relaxed behind the sufferer, holding the hair up with the left hand. When the hollow is visible he presses with his right thumb (nail downwards) three times in and simultaneously up. This treatment can be repeated, if necessary, after an hour or so.

To free yourself of anxiety of any kind — for instance, before tooth extraction — sit very relaxed with your fingers slightly curled. Now with the tip of the thumb press the side of the middle finger on the level of the nail-root and hold it strongly for seven seconds. Once you know the specific point, you do both hands at the same time.

To summarise: The etheric body of our solar system is a whole, comprising planets, humanity and all existing living organisms. The etheric body is the mould upon which the physical body is cast. It consists of a light net of pure energy receiving and passing on life-force. With every act and every thought man affects the inflowing life-force and by its transmission influences the lower kingdoms in nature.

Through this etheric framework the dense physical body is maintained. It can be compared with the circulatory system, as blood flows through arteries and veins, so flows cosmic energy through the etheric body.

As soon as mankind has reached a certain level in evolution, the use of coloured light will help in elimination and building up. Stimulation through music will come into use, dissonances for breaking and shattering; and harmony for building up. Not as it is today on an emotional or mental level, but through knowledge of the sounds of the Rays. Electricity will also be applied for vivication, as we use the sun today.

Disease has its source in disharmony between individuality and personality and affects the etheric body. In this, the Aquarian Age, we will take a step ahead in etheric consciousness and by the end of this century the lowest part of the etheric body will be visible to most people.

More Group Relaxations

Try and find the absolutely ideal position for your relaxation, it does not matter how long you wriggle around, but do find what is right. Right means that it should be so inviting you can think of nothing better than to just be calm and limp, and deeply comfortable for the next hour.

This easy, lovely position will be enhanced if you are also completely at ease inwardly. Looking forward, feeling the peacefulness of this room, feeling completely free, no expectation, no conflict, you look forward to just being yourself. The ideal position includes your tongue, the looseness and limpness of your tongue, so spend a few moments concentrating on your tongue, feel how it is becoming very soft, very broad, lying in the bottom of your mouth, the tip is touching very gently the inner part of the lower gums. The moment your tongue is relaxed, the chin and the jaw relax too, they just cannot help it. and the whole face will follow; you try it.

With every breath . . shallow breathing . . normal breathing, there is no effort . . you sink just a little more deeply down into your blanket. Every breath holds the thought of calmness . . breathe in the calmness and you breathe out calmness into your body . . and through it the body starts to relax more . . It becomes more flexible, always more and more prepared to relax, and before we go and start relaxation proper, you try and tell yourself that you will not go to sleep straight away, you will try and follow the instructions, so that you will get the maximum benefits out of this hour. But, if you should feel terribly drowsy, then just give in, do not try and force it, otherwise you won't be able to relax.

Your eyes being closed, your sight is already turned inwards, one of the most important senses is turned inwards . . One by one you will turn the other senses inwards too, so that you will be completely detached from the outside ready to work from within . . You are first quite aware of the touch, the contact between your body and the ground. Go over your body and feel where you can sense this contact . . back of the head . . the shoulders . . back . . buttocks . . legs . . heels . . and your arms and hands wherever they touch the ground . . You feel the blanket, very light . . warm . . comforting . . and you are conscious of all this outer sense, as though you would make a mental gesture taking it inwards . . take it to the centre of the brain and leave it there . . It will be easy to take your sense of smell and taste from without to within . . to the centre of the brain . . Only your hearing is directed to the outside . . but gradually as you relax more and more, and also with the mental picture, the mental effort to cut the sense as much as possible, you will take the hearing too, to the inside leaving just enough to hear the words which will guide you . . Whatever other sounds may reach you, will not disturb you in the least . . Those guiding words will be all that you will respond to . .

Already your body is very limp, very relaxed, starting to be very peaceful, and it will be quite easy to follow part by part . .

Right palm relax . . right palm relax . . thumb relax . . second finger . . third finger . . fourth finger . . little finger . . go there with our mind and ease out the tension, right wrist relax . . right wrist . . forearm . . elbow . . upper arm relax . . upper arm relax . . go through it with your mind as you relax it . . from within . . deeply . . right shoulder . . right armpit . . right down the right side of your waist . . right hip . . right hip relax . . right thigh, go through the right thigh to the knee . . right knee . . calf relax . . calf relax . . shin . . right ankle . . right ankle relax . . heel . . let it flow through the whole sole of the foot . . and the last tension goes from your right side through the toes . . big toe . . second . . third . . fourth . . and the fifth . . the whole right side of your body . .

162

the whole right side of your body is relaxed . .   very relaxed
  . ,   go to the left palm . .   left palm . .   feel how limp
it is   . .   left palm relax . .   thumb . .   flow through it
  . .   thumb   relax . .   second   finger . .   third . .
fourth . .   do not hurry, take your time . .   little finger
  . .   the   whole   hand   is   utterly   relaxed . .   left   wrist
relax . .   forearm . .   forearm   relax . .   left   elbow
  . .   upper arm . .   shoulder . .   the whole left arm is
heavy and relaxed . .   left armpit . .   right down the left
side   to   the   waist . .   and   the   left   hip . .   left   hip
relax . .   left thigh . .   left thigh relax from inside . .
right down through the knee . .   knee relax . .   knee relax
  . .   left calf . .   shin relax . .   left ankle . .   left heel
  . .   and let it flow through the sole of the foot to the toes
  . .   through the toes . .   big toe . .   second . .   third
  . .   fourth . .   fifth . .   the   whole   left   side   of   your
body . .   the   whole   left   side   of   your   body   is   completely
relaxed . .   completely   relaxed . .   the   whole   spine   from
the head right down . .   down . .   down . .   down . .
into   the   very   coccyx . .   buttocks   relax . .   right   side
  . .   left side . .   all the muscles in your back are limp
now . .   the back is very flat . .   relaxed . .   right shoulder . .   left shoulder . .   back of the neck . .   back of the
neck . .   let the tension go from the skin behind your ears
  . .   right side . .   left side . .   let it go . .   be very
limp . .   back of the head relax . .   back of the head
relax . .   scalp relax . .   scalp relax . .   right ear . .
right temple . .   glide over your forehead relaxing it . .   to
the left temple . .   and the left ear . .   very relaxed . .
soft . .   and very tender . .   relax the point between your
eyebrows . .   right eyebrow . .   left eyebrow . .   both
eyes are relaxed . .   eyelids heavy and relaxed . .   eyeballs
soft . .   sinking . .   sinking deeper . .   deeper into their
sockets . .   right cheek relax . .   left cheek relax . .
bridge of the nose . .   right nostril . .   left nostril . .
your upper lip is perfectly soft . .   the lower lip . .   chin
  . .   jaw . .   relaxing even further now . .   your whole
face is warm and open . .   smooth . .   serene . .   so
relaxed . .   it all feels so good . .   throat relax . .
throat relax . .   right collarbone . .   right side of the
chest . .   left collarbone . .   left side of the chest . .
the whole chest is flat . .   expanding . .   flat . .   relaxed

. . diaphragm relax . . diaphragm relax . . abdomen relax . . your whole body . . the whole body is soft . . expanded . . very light . . very open . . completely peaceful . . your brain is relaxed . . you cannot think . . open and relaxed . . inwardly you are deeply relaxed . . open . . soft, relaxed . . only peacefulness is in you and flows through you . . deep peace . . deep peace . . peace fills every cell . . every part of you is peace . . peace . . peace . . great peace . . peace . . peace . . peace . . peace . . peace . . peace peace . .

Silence for twenty minutes.

Wake up . . awake . . wake up . . but remain perfectly still and relaxed . . try and remember . . did you sleep . . did you dream . . or what were your thoughts . . go over them . . check it for a moment or two . . most of you will find that you feel completely at ease . . very . . very harmonious . . very light . . and somehow ever so far removed from your everyday . . and it is a very good feeling . . thoroughly good . . it is not only a feeling of lightness, but a feeling of tremendous freedom, as though you would suddenly be able to breathe ever so more lightly . . and everything is so light in you that it is absolutely easy to inwardly hear the heart beat . . try to pick it up in the heart itself . . try to pick it up in your left foot . . if your body is properly relaxed the blood can circulate so freely, nothing hampers the flow of it . . nothing hampers the flow of nervous energy . . your whole body is relaxed . . open and free . . really free and light . . and one by one you will now turn your senses from the inside back to the outside to prepare you for the rest of your day . . when you go out, go back to your work, or to your respective recreational occupations. First the sense of taste, then smell returns, then make a gesture, take it from the centre of your brain and switch it to the outside. Your hearing is also turning to the outside now and you listen and pick up any sounds that you may hear, let them come to you, and nothing is grating or irritating, everything is so easy and light . . now the touch . . the sense of touch returns, you are again conscious of the contact between your body and the floor, and the blanket which covers you . . only the sense of sight is still shut, your eyes are still shut, but there is this more and more pronounced feeling of inner well-being, now you start to breathe a little more deliberately, stretching your breath, lengthening your breath . . and with every inhaling you take in prana and as you exhale, let it spread through the body, once more take it in, and this time take it directly to your solar plexus and exhaling, spread it from there and it travels to the toes and to the tips of the fingers . . everywhere and gives you fresh vitality and somehow a joy with which you look forward to the rest of the day, and the other days that will follow. Keep it up for a few moments, conscious . . joyful . . breathing.

Then you move your toes and you wriggle your fingers, hands, and only now do you allow your sight to return outwards, you open your eyes, blink a little, and you get used to the light, and for this last moment you just savour and enjoy the peacefulness.

And then you stretch out, and stretch with joy, stretch with pleasure, and feel thoroughly content, and thoroughly confident and when you are ready you sit up, and look forward to the next item on the agenda.

Relaxation
Inhale, go down through the spine as if you were in it, from the crown down to the coccyx and stay a bit there, and exhale and come up again to the crown, just through the spine . . inhale down . . hold . . and exhale up to the crown . . Inhale down . . exhale up . . repeat this a few times with your own tempo, it has to be easy and without effort . .

Remember you are here of your own free will, and you are completely free . . if you prefer to sleep or follow your own train of thought, you are welcome to it, but naturally your greatest success will be if you follow the suggestions. Remember, to relax is to be easy, to be passive, to let go . . will does not come into it . .

I will suggest parts of the body where you go with your mind . . wherever the mind goes, there goes your consciousness, and that part is immediately relaxed through the consciousness . .

This is how it works . .   Place the tip of the tongue behind your lower front teeth, part your teeth slightly and let the lips just touch . .   so you will not get a dry throat through open mouth breathing . .   you withdraw your senses . .   As you exhale you go deeper . .   and deeper into yourself . .   you go deeper and deeper into yourself . .   deeper and deeper into yourself . .

Withdraw the sense of smell from your nose . .   withdraw it into the middle of your brain . .   Your eyes are closed . .   the eyes deep . .   deep in the sockets and the eyelids very soft . .   very, very soft . .   just falling over the eyes . .   there is no pressure . .   there is only ease . .   that ease will prevent flickering . .   You do not specially strain your eyes to look up or down . .   let the eyes turn where they want to turn . .   do not use any force . .

Then you withdraw the sense of touch . .   You know wherever you touch your body with the tip of a pin you will feel it . .   wherever you feel there are nerves, so your body is completely covered and traversed by nerves . .   it is said that we have a hundred thousand miles of nerves and practically the same amount of blood vessels . .   so you turn your sense of touch inwards that you feel what is going on in the body . .

You withdraw your sense of hearing . .   leaving only a fraction . .   just enough to hear my voice . .   but it should rather come from far away . .   try not to listen to me . .   just hear me . .   follow very leisurely the suggestions . .   it does not matter if you miss out here and there . .   as long as you are very passive . .

Now you withdraw more, you go even deeper . .   and deeper . .   and you hear the blood rush in your ears . .   and you feel the action in your body . .   a sort of humming vibration . .   you realise that every part in your body is active . .   because every moment . .   every split second in your life . .   your body is functioning . .   cells are giving off waste matter . .   and new material is being brought to it . .   and all the time there is action in the body, and it goes into astronomical numbers . .

Now you feel your throat . .   throat relax . .   throat relax . .   make it very easy . .   feel the expansion in the

throat and be conscious of the breath going in and out . . it
should be a sheer pleasure . . tongue relax . . tongue
relax . . lips relax . . lips relax . . nose relax . .
nose relax . . right temple relax . . right temple relax
 . . left temple relax . . left temple relax . . forehead
relax . . forehead relax . . right cheek relax . . right
cheek relax . . left cheek relax . . left cheek relax . .
now your whole face is utterly relaxed . . and you can feel
the smoothness of your skin . . it is a delightful feeling and
you feel lovely . . and beautiful . .

Scalp relax . . scalp relax . . back of the head relax
 . . back of the head relax . . brain relax . . brain
relax . . right ear relax . . right ear relax . . left ear
relax . . left ear relax . . now your head feels wonderfully cool and easy and there is only ease . . no tension . .
no stress . . only ease . . it is an exquisite feeling, and
you can't help smiling . . chest relax . . chest relax . .
your chest gets very flat . . flatter and flatter . . so flat
the abdomen comes out a bit . . ribs relax . . ribs relax
 . . abdomen relax . . abdomen relax . .

In the middle of your body . . near your spine . . you
have the most sensitive part in you . . the solar plexus . .
any emotion, positive or negative, first registers there . . you
know where you have butterflies . . where you have tension
 . . so now imagine you have a very tight belt, so tight that
it is uncomfortable then you open it and let it go . . you
have that wonderful feeling of expansion . . and the last bit
of tension in the solar plexus is gone . .

Now you feel your breathing . . and you are an onlooker,
it is really as if someone else would breathe you . . you can
just feel it go in . . and out . . it is fully automatic, and
it is as if you had nothing whatever to do with it . . Then
you go with your mind deep . . deep in the right shoulder
 . . right shoulder relax . . right shoulder relax . .
right upper arm relax . . right upper arm relax . . right
elbow relax . . right elbow relax . . right forearm relax
 . . right forearm relax . . right wrist relax . . right
wrist relax ..

And now you feel the centre of the right palm . . now as
your attention is there you feel the blood tingling . . and
as you feel it . . it gets stronger . . and stronger . .

till it is a strong vibration . . and even stronger till it is a strong pulsation . . and you can feel the blood pulsate in the right hand . . and you can feel the blood pulsate in the right thumb . . and you can feel the blood pulsate in the right forefinger . . and you can feel the blood pulsate in the right middle finger . . and you can feel the blood pulsate in the right ring finger . . and you can feel the blood pulsate in the right little finger . . now you can feel the pulsation in the whole right hand . . getting stronger . . and stronger . . and it spreads over the whole right arm . . and for a moment . . just lie there and enjoy the feeling of your blood circulation . .

Now go with your mind deep . . deep into the left shoulder . . left shoulder relax . . left shoulder relax . . left upper arm relax . . left upper arm relax . . left elbow relax . . left elbow relax . . left forearm relax . . left forearm relax . . left wrist relax . . left wrist relax . . and now you can feel the tingling of the blood in the left palm . . it gets stronger and you can feel that strong vibration . . then you feel the strong pulsation . . and you can feel the blood pulsating in the whole left hand . . and you feel the blood pulsate in the left thumb . . and you feel the blood pulsate in the left forefinger . . and you feel the blood pulsate in the left middle finger . . and you feel the blood pulsate in the left ring finger . . and you feel the pulsation of the blood in the left little finger . . and you can feel the strong pulsation in the whole left hand . . and in the whole left arm . . now you can feel the blood pulsate in both of your arms . .

From deep . . deep within you . . you go to the right hip . . right hip relax . . right hip relax . . right thigh relax . . right thigh relax . . right knee relax . . right knee relax . . right calf relax . . right calf relax . . right ankle relax . . right ankle relax . . right foot relax . . right foot relax . . now again you feel the centre of your right foot . . and you immediately feel the tingling of the blood in it . . and it gets stronger . . and stronger . . till it is a strong vibration . . and even stronger . . till it is a strong pulsation . . and you can feel the blood pulsate through your whole foot . . and then through the whole right leg . .

And from deep . . deep within you . . you feel the left hip . . left hip relax . . left hip relax . . left thigh relax . . left thigh relax . . left knee relax . . left knee relax . . left calf relax . . left calf relax . . left ankle relax . . left ankle relax . . left foot relax . . left foot relax . . and you feel the tingling in the left footsole . . getting stronger . . being a strong vibration . . getting stronger . . till you feel a very strong pulsation . . and you can feel the blood pulsate through the whole left foot . . and then through the left leg . . and you can feel the blood pulsate through both your legs now every part in you is utterly relaxed . .

You feel wonderfully serene . . contented . . and happy . . and to get rid of all the frustrations . . of all the heartaches . . of all the sorrows . . all the worries . . all the depressions . . I give to you the suggestion of Divine Peace . . and you feel the Divine Peace filling every cell of your body, and as it fills . . all the negativeness is pushed out . . where there is Divine Peace . . there is no sorrow . . there is no hatred . . or frustration . . Divine Peace fills you . . Divine Peaces fills you . . Divine Peace fills you . .

Repeat Divine Peace fills you thirty to sixty times . . Silence twenty minutes.

End ritual.